Communicating at the End of Life

Finding Magic in the Mundane

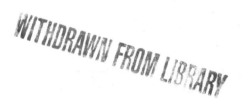

LEA's Series on Personal Relationships
Steve Duck, Series Editor

For more information on LEA titles, please contact Lawrence Erlbaum Associates, Publishers, at www.erlbaum.com

Communicating at the End of Life

Finding Magic in the Mundane

Elissa Foster
San José State University

LAWRENCE ERLBAUM ASSOCIATES, PUBLISHERS
2007   **Mahwah, New Jersey**   **London**

Copyright © 2007 by Lawrence Erlbaum Associates, Inc.
  All rights reserved. No part of this book may be reproduced in any
  form, by photostat, microform, retrieval system, or any other means,
  without prior written permission of the publisher.

Lawrence Erlbaum Associates, Inc., Publishers
10 Industrial Avenue
Mahwah, New Jersey 07430
www.erlbaum.com

Cover design by Kathryn Houghtaling Lacey

Library of Congress Cataloging-in-Publication Data

Foster, Elissa. Communicating at the end of life : Finding magic in the
  mundane.
      p. cm.
    Includes bibliographical references and index.
ISBN 978-0-8058-5566-1 (cloth)
ISBN 978-0-8058-5567-8 (pbk.)
ISBN 978-1-4106-1545-9 (e book)
1. Hospice care. 2. Volunteer workers in terminal care. 3. Interpersonal
  communication. I. Title.
R726.8F68   2006
362.17′56—dc22   2006013774
                                                        CIP

Books published by Lawrence Erlbaum Associates are printed on acid-
free paper, and their bindings are chosen for strength and durability.

Printed in the United States of America
10 9 8 7 6 5 4 3 2 1

*Dedicated to the memory
of Margaret Ella Ward
1919–1994*

Contents

Part II: Entering the Country of the Dying

Part III: Communication as Improvisation: Learning How to "Be There" for People at the End of Life

Series Foreword

Steve Duck
Series Editor

Since its inception the Personal Relationships series from Lawrence Erlbaum Associates has sought to review the progress in the academic work on relationships with respect to a broad array of issues and to do so in an accessible manner that also illustrates its *practical* value. The LEA series already includes books intended to pass on the accumulated scholarship to the next generation of students and to those who deal with relationship issues in the broader world beyond the academy, including issues of life cycle, networks, sexual behavior, relating difficulty, affairs, nonverbal communication, and maintaining relationships. The series thus not only comprises monographs and other academic resources exemplifying the multidisciplinary nature of this area, but also books suitable for use in the growing numbers of courses on relationships and in the growing number of professions that recognize the importance of relationship issues in their work.

The series has the goal of providing a comprehensive and current survey of theory and research in personal relationships through the careful analysis of the problems encountered and solved, yet it also considers the systematic application of that work in a practical context. These resources not only are intended to be comprehensive assessments of progress on particular "hot" and relevant topics, but also have already shown that they are significant influences on the future directions and development of the study of personal relationships and application of its insights. Although each volume is well centered, authors all attempt to place the respective topics in the broader context of other research on relationships and within a range of wider disciplinary traditions. The series already offers incisive and forward-looking reviews and also demonstrates the broader implications of relationships for the range of disciplines from which the research originates. Collectively the volumes include practical application, original studies, reviews of relevant theory and research, and new approaches to the understanding of personal relationships both in themselves and within the context of broader theories of family process, social psychology, and communication.

Reflecting the diverse composition of personal relationship study, readers in numerous disciplines—social psychology, communication, sociology, family studies, developmental psychology, clinical psychology, personality, counseling, women's studies, gerontology, and others—will find valuable and insightful perspectives in the series both within and outside their own discipline.

Apart from the academic scholars who research the dynamics and processes of relationships, there are many other people whose work takes them up against the operation of relationships in the real world. For such people as nurses, the police, teachers, therapists, lawyers, drug and alcohol counselors, marital counselors, the priesthood, and those who take care of the elderly, the sick or the dying, a number of issues routinely arise concerning the ways in which relationships affect the people whom they serve and guide. Examples are the role of loneliness in illness and the ways to circumvent it, the complex impact of family and peer relationships on a drug-dependent's attempts to give up the drug, the role of playground unpopularity on a child's learning, the issues involved in dealing with the relational side of chronic illness and imminent death, the management of conflict in marriage, the establishment of good rapport between physicians and seriously ill patients, the support of the bereaved, the correction of violent styles of behavior in dating or marriage, and even the relationships formed between jurors in extended trials as these may influence a jury's decisions. Each of these is a problem that may confront some of the aforementioned professionals as part of their daily concerns and each demonstrates the far-reaching influences of relationship processes on much else in life that is presently theorized independently of relationship considerations.

Elissa Foster's elegant, lucid, and appealing contribution to this series deals with the relational context of caring for the dying and terminally ill. Based on the insights gained from a painful personal experience, and her decision to become involved in hospice care, her book illuminates the processes both from the perspective of the independent hospice care-worker and also from the perspective of the immediate family and the patient herself. The author introduces herself as a human being who has experienced loss and wishes to help others as they also deal with it. But she is also an accomplished ethnographer and is able to offer not only humane but also theoretically driven insight into the whole complex process. The chapters are written extraordinarily well and are very engaging. The humanity of the author comes across as well as complexity and insight that she offers in analysis of the issues that are described in the book. There is a very clear presentation of the issues that are involved in caring for the dying and also well depicted are the surrounding issues of the life that the person is leaving. The author successfully draws us into this narrative and also does a certain amount of self-disclosure that helps us to understand some of the issues that might affect us if we were in the same position, which is an increasingly likely long-term possibility for us all.

The book is a truly winning contribution to the series notwithstanding its initially forbidding topic. The reader finishes the book feeling enlightened, saddened, informed, and yet ultimately uplifted and moved. It is an important book.

Preface

As human beings, we are undeniably mortal, and for that reason, communication at the end of life is a subject that is significant to all of us. In addition to its general significance, the topic of this book will attract some readers who have a professional interest as health care practitioners or academics, and most readers will have personal reasons for wanting to know more about communication at the end of life. Many readers may turn to a book like this one because they have cared for someone who is dying, are facing the prospect of taking on such a role, or because they themselves are facing a limited amount of time to live and would like to know more about hospice. My own involvement with hospice began when I recognized that despite having studied interpersonal communication and relationships for many years, I had very little experience and a great deal of anxiety when it came to communicating with someone who was facing the end of his or her life. In truth, it was the most difficult thing I could imagine doing, and also something that I wanted to be able to do well, which is why I turned to hospice to help me overcome my fears and provide me with an opportunity to respond confidently, compassionately, and completely to those who are dying.

Because I recognize that this topic is of interest to a variety of people who come from a range of backgrounds, professions, and academic disciplines, I recognize also that readers may have a range of expectations about how this book will be presented. For that reason, I would like to explain a little about how this book was researched, how it is organized, and how I invite readers to approach it. The format of this book is dictated, in part, by my training as a narrative ethnographer. Ethnographic research is grounded in the conviction that we can best understand social behaviors and meanings by directly engaging with the contexts in which they occur. Ethnographers are concerned with meaning as embedded in the practices, language, contexts, ideas, and events of a culture, as well as the subjective meanings of the individual within that culture. The stories in this book were generated through 12 months of pre-fieldwork study, 18 months of participation as a hospice volunteer, and three sets of interviews conducted at 6-month intervals with a panel of volunteers. The story of my own volunteering experience was generated through methods associated with autoethnography, which involved both ongoing field notes related to my experience, and later, a rigorous process of narrative writing aimed at capturing the details of interaction and relationship that were most relevant to this study of end-of-life communication. A comprehensive description and rationale for my method are provided in the Appendix, and I encourage readers to turn to this discussion either as an introduction to the study or as curiosity motivates you to do so.

At this juncture, I would like to emphasize that as a narrative ethnographer, my goal was to directly engage with the activities and culture of hospice through the experience of volunteering, to embrace its complexity, and to convey through narrative writing the qualities and concrete particulars of my experience and that of the other volunteers. As I experienced what it was like to be a hospice volunteer and talk to other volunteers, my goal was to uncover and adequately represent practices and meanings that were specific to this place, this time, and these people. Much of the scholarly work of this study consisted of analyzing hundreds of pages of notes and transcripts, identifying the most relevant or "telling" elements in relation to the central purpose of the book, and composing the results into a form that allowed the richness of the experiences to shine through. The stories that were generated through this research process are the foundation, and, I believe, the most important contribution of the book.

The emphasis on stories should pose no problem for those who are reading primarily to understand what hospice is like, the role of the volunteers, and how the volunteers communicated with patients at the end of life. What has been challenging for me is how to integrate into the stories the kinds of cultural and social analysis that are expected of a scholarly book. My solution has been to offer, wherever possible, theories, facts, background information, and explanation as part of the stories. Periodically, I offer more extensive conceptual discussions at the end of the chapters as reflections on questions that are raised by the stories. For some readers, these will be less relevant, and I assure those readers that the stories do not suffer in the absence of the academic reflections if you should choose to skip them (although the same is not true in the reverse). For other readers, the stories will call out for explanation and framing within the ongoing conversations of the communication discipline, both within interpersonal and health communication scholarship. I note here that although there are a growing number of scholars working in this area, there is as yet no body of literature or core theory that addresses the end-of-life context in terms of interpersonal relationships. I gratefully acknowledge the health and interpersonal communication scholars whose work I cite in the pages that follow, and I also preview my analysis by admitting my tendency to return to "first principles" of interpersonal communication—the content and relational levels of messages, dialogue and dialectics, and intersubjectivity—to help explain what I observed in the relationships between hospice volunteers and patients.

One challenge of taking a narrative ethnographic approach to my topic is that the stories I present will be far richer in their implications than my analysis could possibly address in the scope of this book. This means that some readers, even from my home discipline of communication, will no doubt be disappointed that I did not address some aspects of the stories that are important to them, or that I did not spend enough time on some issues while devoting extensive time to others. That is a burden of authorship that I am willing to bear because I recognize that stories are complex in the ways that life is complex, and, as such, they will provoke responses and ideas in readers that I did not necessarily see in the same way—which is as it should be.

What I do offer in the academic reflections throughout the book, and in various asides throughout the stories, are insights into hospice and the end-of-life context from my own particular standpoint as an interpersonal communication scholar who focuses on issues of health and well-being. This standpoint implies several things. First, that I will focus on the messages that are sent and received both by the participants in the study—that is, the other volunteers I interviewed—and by the people who inhabit the stories: patients, caregivers, hospice workers, and others. Second, I am particularly concerned with the aspects of communication that have to do with relationships. For me, that implies as much emphasis on the implicit aspects of communication as it does on the words and ideas that are exchanged. The ethnographic methods I used to conduct the study allow for a deeper exploration of these implicit, relational aspects of communication than do many other methods. Specifically, the active participation demanded by ethnography combined with the introspective processes of autothenographic narrative writing together constitute a powerful method of learning through living. Many of the insights we take for granted in our daily interactions are significant to our process of making meaning, but are almost impossible to study from the perspective of an objective observer. As I delve into the more conceptual and theoretical discussions of relational communication, I recognize that these insights (while fascinating to me) may be less relevant to other kinds of readers, so I have also tried to incorporate explicit links to practical implications for volunteers, patients, families, and clinicians. This brings me to the third implication of my interests as an author: My interests in health and wellness, and my training as an ethnographer, make it impossible for me to discuss relationships without considering the contexts in which those relationships are enacted. In this case, hospice impacts the relationships between volunteers and patients both as an organization with rules and norms like any other, and also as a philosophy of care that has an associated set of values, principles, and language.

Before previewing the parts of the book, I offer a note of explanation about my use of hospice terms to describe the relationships and experiences of the volunteers; particularly, the word *patients*. Although it resists the biomedical model of care, hospice is still primarily understood to be a medical service; thus the term *patient* persists as the descriptor for those who receive hospice services. The term *patient* casts the receiver of hospice services into a passive role on the receiving, and thus lower, end of a biomedical hierarchy, and so it is certainly open to critique for that reason. However, it would be inauthentic of me to substitute a different term in this book—for example, *client, resident,* or *recipient*—simply to avoid warranted scrutiny and critique. Nevertheless, I would like to preempt some of that critique by explaining how the phrase *my patient* (which to some may sound additionally proprietary) operated for the volunteers.

Although we did not have patients in the same way that the clinical members of the team did, to suggest that volunteers call patients something different from how they are referred to by the rest of the hospice team is problematic. Not only is it very difficult to come up with an adequate descriptor (I've tried!), to use a different term also suggests that the volunteers are not, in fact, contributing to patient care to the same degree or in the same way that other members of the clinical team are. It should also be noted that the term *my patient* was used far more in this research than it would normally be used by a volunteer. When communicating in hospice contexts—in patient notes, support meetings, or with our coordinators—volunteers mostly referred to patients by their names. In their interviews with me, in the interests of confidentiality, rather than say he, she, or (as one volunteer put it)"this person," the volunteers adopted the generic term *my patient*. For those who are still concerned that the term *my patient* is problematic because it suggests a hierarchical relationship, I believe the stories in the book will be testament that the volunteers' attitudes toward their patients were neither distanced nor patronizing; rather they reflect the unique and often intimate caring connections that emerged over time. The stories in the book present some other problematic phrases or terms such as *graduating,* when a patient is released from hospice; *passing,* as a euphemism for dying; or *terminal*, to describe a patient's prognosis. These are the actual words used in the interviews or by hospice personnel, and where it does not interrupt the flow of the story, I have tried to indicate problems with the language while recognizing that such language use reveals aspects of our culture (and in some cases the hospice culture) that should be acknowledged.

The book is organized chronologically and follows the course of my involvement with hospice and the phases of the study. The first phase of my research included reading about the history of the hospice movement, making contact with hospice for the first time, and completing the volunteer training program. Part I describes these early contacts with hospice, and provides background and contextual information that will help readers to understand subsequent stories about communication between volunteers and patients. Part II tells the story of my first contact with my patient, Dorothy, and presents stories from the first round of interviews with the other volunteers in my study, which were completed within a few weeks of finishing the hospice training. The emphasis in Part II is on the adjustments the volunteers made as we entered the world of hospice and the worlds of our patients. Part III presents stories from my ongoing visits with Dorothy, as well as stories from the second round of interviews that were conducted 4 months after the training. The emphasis in Part III is on the importance of improvisation and finding balance within our roles as volunteers, and particularly how to be fully present for our patients and their family members. Part IV addresses how the volunteers coped with the deaths of our patients, and what we learned from the experience of volunteering. I conclude by drawing together implications from the study as they relate to communicating at the end of life in hospice.

ACKNOWLEDGMENTS

First, I must acknowledge the extraordinary generosity of the volunteers who participated in this study; this book would not exist without their willingness and ability to describe their insights so that others could benefit from them. Norma Sanchez was an unwavering source of enthusiasm and support for my own journey as a hospice volunteer, and I hope this book will stand as a tribute to her expansive heart and her dedication to her work. I also wish to acknowledge the Center for Hospice, Palliative Care, and End-of-Life Studies at the University of South Florida for its support of my research through its Pilot Studies Grant Program, as well as LifePath Hospice and Palliative Care. May your important work continue to grow and influence how we care for people at the end of life.

This book would not exist without the unwavering and dedicated support that I received from members of the faculty in the Department of Communication Studies at the University of South Florida, particularly my advisor and dissertation director, Art Bochner. Before I began my doctoral program, he challenged me to engage in passionate scholarship, and I have never looked back. I extend many thanks to Ken Cissna, Eric Eisenberg, Carolyn Ellis, and Larry Polivka who provided the perfect blend of inspiration and critical insight.

I gratefully acknowledge Steve Duck for his visionary and tireless work within the field of communication studies and for taking the time to talk to a beginning scholar about her work, then encouraging (and reading and suggesting and editing) that work toward this final outcome. Having my book in his relationships book series is an extraordinary honor. At Lawrence Erlbaum Associates, I thank Linda Bathgate for her kind support, Karin Bates and Sara Scudder for working on the production of the book, and the anonymous reviewers who provided valuable feedback as the book developed.

My warmest thanks to my colleagues, too numerous to mention, who have nourished me with a thousand remarkable conversations over the years. To my parents, Bill and Barbara Foster, and my entire personal cheering squad in Australia (Jo and Morgan, Ande and Su, Barb, Jo, and Sally), who urged me on from 15,000 miles away, as well as those a little closer (Yasmin and Christine)—I thank you. Finally, to my friend and partner, Jay Baglia, who was present through the living and the writing, the frustration and the inspiration: You've supported me in a thousand ways, physically, emotionally, and intellectually, with your great cooking, your insightful readings, and your love. I can not imagine making this life journey without you. You are the best one of all.

—*Elissa Foster*

PART I

Hospice as a Context of Health Care and Interpersonal Communication

An important aspect of narrative storytelling is establishing the character and voice of the narrator. In this case, in order for the reader to understand, interpret, and critique the story I tell about hospice, it is necessary for me to reveal the aspects of my character and history that contributed to the events of the story, and to my perspective on those events. In addition, just as setting the scene is an essential part of narrative, establishing the context for the study is an important part of ethnographic writing. In Part I, I invest some time in describing the origins of my involvement with hospice as well as the origins of the hospice movement, and some of the organizational features of hospice that are essential to understanding the context in which the relationships between volunteers and patients were initiated and unfolded.

In chapter 1, I describe my first face-to-face contact with hospice, I provide a rationale for integrating my personal story with the academic reflections that occur throughout the book, and I close the chapter by defining hospice as a social movement, a type of organization, and as the particular organization, LifePath Hospice and Palliative Care, in which I conducted the study. In chapter 2, I describe the aspects of the volunteer training that related most closely to the communication between volunteers and patients, and to the nature of the volunteer role within hospice. Throughout my description of the training, I periodically provide some observations from hospice and end-of-life research that link the content of the training to the literature. The voice I employ in chapter 2 tends to privilege an academic perspective, mostly because without experience as a point of reference for the information I received, my understanding of the training was

1

framed by what I had read about hospice. I conclude Part I with reflections on the volunteer training and my perspective as I stood on the threshold of meeting a hospice patient.

1

Beginnings

AM I READY?

It's a perfect day in Tampa, early December; the sun is warm but not hot, the breeze is cool but not cold. I park my car under the oak trees that surround the single-story building and stride toward the glass doors. Inside, I hesitate and hover a few feet behind a tall, middle-aged woman who is chatting cheerfully with the receptionist. The woman leans over the counter, obviously comfortable in this environment and, by comparison, I feel every bit the outsider that I am. Suddenly self-conscious, I scan the small foyer in an attempt to appear relaxed. It is an inviting space, with comfortable seats and a wealth of pamphlets—a blend of business office, hospital reception, and private doctor's waiting room. The space is welcoming, but the signs on the doors and the employees' identification badges signal that I have entered a medical environment. Still, I'm not as intimidated as I might be in a hospital or doctor's office, and I remind myself that I'm here for a good reason.

"May I help you?" the receptionist asks as I step into the space recently vacated by the cheerful visitor. The receptionist appears to be in her early 70s, older than I expected.

"Yes, I hope so," I begin. "I wanted some information about becoming a volunteer."

"Let me see if someone's available to talk with you," she says, turning away from me to pick up her phone.

"I don't really need to talk to anyone," I begin, fruitlessly trying to stop her from calling. "Don't you have a packet?" I trail off as someone picks up her call somewhere in the building.

She turns back to me, briefly, with the phone to her ear. "What's your name, dear?"

"Elissa Foster," I reply before she speaks into the phone again.

She completes the call and then turns to face me and says, "Norma Sanchez is the volunteer coordinator. She'll be out to see you in a few minutes."

"Okay," I reply. "Thank you."

I had intended this visit to be quick, anonymous, and easily reversible if I decide to back out. Now, it seems I must meet someone and give an account of myself. Can't they just give me some printed information that I can read in private? I don't know if I'm ready to commit, and I'm unsure of my ability to say no if I feel pressure to sign up.

Looking around, my gaze is drawn to a permanent display on the wall—a sculptured metal tree with small brass leaves surrounding the branches. As I draw closer, I see names and dates commemorating loved ones and celebrating the work of the organization. On the wall beside the tree are more plaques and awards; I wonder about the faces and stories behind the names. I pick up an in-house newsletter. The feature story describes how one volunteer became involved; there is a Q & A section inside and, on the back, a section titled "Want to know more?" I realize that this question is directed to me.

I hear an internal door opening onto the foyer and slip the newsletter into my briefcase.

"Hello, Elissa?" I hear a friendly and vivacious voice behind me.

When I turn, an attractive, bright-eyed woman in her 40s is walking toward me. She smiles broadly as she extends her hand and I can't help but smile back.

"I'm Norma Sanchez. I'm a volunteer coordinator here at LifePath Hospice. Why don't we find somewhere to talk?" Norma ushers me through the door from which she just emerged. "Do you have time?"

"Sure." My pulse quickens as I realize that this is the beginning of the journey.

We enter a labyrinth of office cubicles and weave swiftly through narrow corridors. I quickly lose my sense of direction. I notice that several employees are wrapping cabinet doors and covering notice boards with Christmas paper and ribbons to look like gifts. The whole space sparkles with color and tinsel.

"We like to decorate for the holidays," Norma informs me with a smile.

"Looks great," I respond, noting the sense of belonging and stewardship communicated by the act of decorating a space. I wonder if people stay in these jobs a long time.

"Did you call and speak to someone?" Norma asks.

"Yes. I called a while ago and requested information. But then, I was going to be in the neighborhood anyway, so I just decided to drop by."

I do not mention that my request for information was never answered. I also gloss over my hectic drive from the north side of town through heavy traffic on the interstate. Still trying to appear casual and unconcerned, I suppress the fact that I drove 15 miles to put myself "in the neighborhood" so I could just "drop by."

Norma introduces me to some of the women in the office. "Elissa is interested in becoming a volunteer."

Amidst a collective murmuring of approval, someone asks, "Do you want to volunteer with patients?"

"Yes, I think so," I reply, and everyone smiles. I'm beginning to enjoy the attention, so I'm also beginning to relax. Norma finds an empty office and we settle in.

"So, tell me about yourself," she takes me by surprise. I expected a prefabricated spiel about hospice and the duties of a volunteer; instead, I'm called to tell a story.

In a few sentences, I describe my work as a researcher and teacher in interpersonal communication and health care. Norma asks questions often, and we quickly move to the topic of my family and my home in Australia.

Then, she asks, "How did you hear about hospice?"

I describe my experiences with another research project that focused on the work of private geriatric care managers. This project introduced me to the field of communication and aging, and the participants I interviewed often mentioned hospice as a medical organization that was exceptionally humane and holistic in its approach.

"So, I developed an academic interest in hospice as well as a personal one," I explain. "I'd like to find out how hospice manages to do what it does—particularly when most of the medical profession isn't good at developing relationships and communicating with patients. From everything I've heard, although hospice is a medical organization, it consistently provides personal care and support to patients and families."

Norma smiles, "Hospice is wonderful and I love working here. It's also true that hospice is an organization like any other. We're not perfect."

I nod quietly. Despite my efforts to be detached and objective, I tend to place hospice and everyone who works here on a pedestal. Perhaps my nervousness stems from this idealized image of hospice work. Norma's observation that hospice is "not perfect" tempers my idealism and reminds me that I have much to learn about the reality of the organization.

"Now, Elissa, I want to ask you a couple of questions that I ask everyone who is interested in volunteering. First, have you had any losses in your life? Not just someone in your life who has died, because there are all kinds of losses—losing a job, a divorce or separation, even the death of a pet can be a significant loss."

When I volunteered for hospitals in the past, the coordinators didn't remember my name from one week to the next, let alone ask about my life and motivations. Although I can imagine some people feeling defensive in response to this question, because of Norma's obvious interest in me and her work with hospice patients, I don't mind talking about painful experiences.

"Well, I was divorced earlier this year," I respond. "It was the right thing to do and I have no regrets, but I miss my husband's family a great deal." Even as I say this to Norma, I recognize that, for me, talking about being divorced is more embarrassing than painful.

Noticing my discomfort, Norma says, "I've been there, too. It's okay."

"And I suppose I also deal with being away from my family."

"I can hardly imagine; you're so far from home!" Norma exclaims. "You said that all your family is in Australia?"

I nod. "And we're very close, even though we live on different continents."

"Do you have grandparents or older relatives there? Or are they deceased?"

I take a breath. "Actually, my only living grandparent, my grandmother, died soon after I moved to the United States. That's probably the most important reason for why I came."

When I left Australia I knew my grandmother was near the end of her life. She had been diagnosed with lymphoma 18 months earlier, and I had sought information from my own general practitioner about her prognosis. My doctor described my grandmother's outlook as "not good." In retrospect, I regret that I did not make myself more available to her as she struggled with cancer. She approached her disease in the same tough, no-nonsense way she did everything else. I remember helping her to contact the Cancer Society when she needed a wig, and taking her to and from her appointments, but we never spoke about her feelings, or mine. Although I didn't admit it at the time, I was glad that she never brought it up; that way, I was able to cling to the comfort of my own denial.

In August, when the day came for me to leave for graduate school, I could barely speak to her. I told her that it was very hard to leave and that I loved her very much. When she said, "I know," she communicated so much—that she knew I loved her, that she knew how difficult my decision to leave had been, and that she knew we would not see each other again. I resisted an emotional display because she was her usual, stoic self. I hugged her until she said, "Go now." I left her apartment quickly, crying, hoping that I had said enough, fearing that I hadn't. I think she planned that to be our last contact, but as we pulled away in the car to go

to the airport, she walked out to the front gate to wave me off. I blew kisses out the back window until she disappeared from view.

When the phone call came from my mother in early December, I was shocked. I didn't expect Grandma to die so soon. I told myself she would celebrate her birthday in March and this fantasy sheltered me from thinking about her dying at all. Of course, her death would have surprised me no matter when it happened, because I never allowed myself to face the reality of her illness. Whenever I called home and asked to speak to Grandma, I was mystified by the prolonged silence on the line before my mother or father would say gently, "Not tonight." It never occurred to me that she was too weak to talk. Because I did not stay to take care of her, I never saw the way the cancer ravaged her body; I only saw it reflected in my sister's eyes when she told me many months later, "It was horrible. She didn't look like Grandma anymore." I could see how vivid that memory was for my sister, but I had no experience with which to understand what it was like to watch a loved one's body deteriorate to a point beyond recognition. When I remember my Grandma, I have the luxury of seeing her with a straight back, strong arms, and bright eyes, but now I mourn both my grandmother and the opportunities and responsibilities I surrendered when I left to begin graduate school.

"Was your grandmother in hospice?" Norma asks.

"No. I think in Australia hospices are like hospitals—only for people who can't stay at home. My Mum took a leave of absence from her job and was her primary caregiver, though Mum also had a lot of support from my sister and my Dad. Grandma's doctor coordinated her medical care and the community nurses came to the house every day or so. My mother speaks very fondly of the nurse who took care of Grandma. I get the impression that it was a very important relationship for my mother and for my grandmother, too. They became very close."

"Do you wish that you'd been there for your grandmother?" Norma asks.

"I did feel that way for many months. I felt guilty about leaving, especially since I never got to speak to my grandmother again. I also felt like I let my mother down by not being there to help her. It took me a long time to talk about anything to do with Grandma's death. When I was finally ready to hear about it, I wanted to know what it was like, and the story she told me about the last few days of my grandmother's life reassured me, a lot."

My mother told me this story. "It was the last day of the school year and I had planned to attend the end-of-year church service. I had been on leave for weeks, but I wanted to see the students who were graduating, and I also needed the support of the other teachers. Well, I soon saw that Grandma needed me to stay with her, so I called Sheila in the principal's office to say I wouldn't be able to make it to the service. She said, 'It's all right. We understand. You know we'll all be praying for you. The service will be for you and your mother.'

"I was disappointed about missing the service and, after a lifetime of struggle, I wanted to feel close to my mother. You may not know this, but when I first wanted to go to art school, she thought my plan was very frivolous—but she supported me anyway. For some reason, this was on my mind as I came back from talking to Sheila. I also realized that few of the other teachers or my students had ever met Grandma, yet they were sending her their love. So I told her, 'You did a really good thing sending me to art school. I've been able to touch the lives of hundreds of children through the years, and those children are up at the school praying for you right now.'

"She didn't look at me but she quietly said, 'I know.'

"Later that morning, I was giving her a sponge bath and as I stroked her forehead she closed her eyes and said, 'My darling child ....'

"That was the only time she ever called me 'darling.'

"She lost consciousness a little while later and we finally had to take her to the hospital that afternoon. She died the next day."

As my mother told me that story, tears welled in her eyes and her face expressed sadness, strength, and pride. As I tell Norma my mother's story, I am more aware of the reason I am here, and I wonder if my own apparent grief will seem to Norma like an unresolved issue that makes me unsuitable to be a hospice volunteer.

Almost as if she's reading my thoughts, Norma asks, "How do you think that experience has influenced your decision to become a volunteer?"

I struggle to summarize something that has been a complex and hard-won realization for me. "I no longer think about my Grandmother's death only with sadness and regret. My mother's story helps me to understand the meaning of my grandmother's illness in terms of their relationship with each other. In those last moments, my mother and grandmother connected in a way that they hadn't before. They faced death together and, rather than being just a painful and tragic time, those last days were a blessing to them."

"You still miss your grandmother very much, don't you?" Norma asks.

"Yes, I do, but it doesn't hurt as much as it used to," I reply. "The worst thing now is the feeling that I may not respond well to being with someone who is very ill or dying."

I worry that the aspects of my character that led me to deny my grandmother's illness are still there. By becoming a hospice volunteer, I hope to learn how to support a person who is dying. Though I can't go back and rewrite my story, I may not be condemned to relive it.

Norma leans forward, and my gaze is drawn to hers. "Elissa, what you're feeling is very, very common. It's normal to be afraid of death and dying—most people are. That doesn't mean you won't be a good volunteer. The important thing is that you came here; that shows you have a real interest in doing the work. Is anything else worrying you?"

"Well, I didn't have a good experience the last time I was a volunteer." I tell Norma what happened at the last hospital for which I volunteered, how redundant and unneeded I felt, and how I simply stopped going after only 3 months.

"It sounds like they didn't give you anything worthwhile to do," Norma responds, reassuringly. "Let me tell you more about our program. First of all, this is all about you and what you're comfortable with. Second, you will complete 20 hours of training before you ever get asked to see a patient. Third, you choose the type of patient you want to see, whether they're at home or in a nursing home, or if you want to transport patients or not. You elect where you want to work and the times you're available, and we match your interests with the patient's needs.

"We've had some specific requests in the past and we're almost always able to fulfill them. One 57-year-old man asked for someone to play chess with him once a week. We had another patient whose child needed outings. Our patients have a range of diagnoses, physical capabilities, and needs; some are mobile and some are not; some are able to communicate verbally and some are not. Keep an open mind. We care for all kinds of people, of all ages and in all kinds of situations—from the wealthiest CEO to the poorest of the poor. It's important to focus on the patient, not on the environment that you will be in."

Already, my mind is racing into the future, imagining myself in these different situations with patients. I had assumed that hospice patients would be elderly, bed-bound, and in the last weeks of their lives—and this is clearly not the case. I may volunteer for a child who is dying.

"Have you ever had a patient that you couldn't find a volunteer for?" I ask.

"Only one; he was convicted of sexually abusing children. He's out of prison now, but that conviction is a part of his record and we disclose everything to the volunteers so they can make an informed decision. So far, no one has agreed to visit him."

I register a potent combination of shock, revulsion, and unexpected compassion for this man. I imagine him, old, sick, and lonely, longing for human contact and having his need go unanswered. Although I am disgusted by his crime, I object to the idea of him dying alone more than I object to what he did. I also realize that it's easy for me to feel this way when becoming his volunteer is only a hypothetical proposition.

I voice my concerns. "Surely this person, perhaps more than any other, needs someone to talk to and support him at the end of his life?"

Norma shrugs and shakes her head slightly. "You may be right. But volunteers have a right to set their boundaries. I would rather have a volunteer turn down a patient than risk having them visit a patient with mental reservations and moral judgments. The patient will sense if you're uncomfortable. If you are, it's better that you don't see them at all."

Norma continues, "I should also tell you that we would never intentionally send you into a dangerous situation, but there are lots of things you could encounter that distress you. I had one patient who liked pornography and he had explicit pictures of naked women all over the walls of his room. I wouldn't expect a volunteer to go there unless they felt comfortable with that. I did find a male volunteer and, although he said it was shocking at first, he got used to it. The patient was a nice guy—he just happened to like pornography."

This is a lot for me to process, and I decide that I need specifics before my imagination goes completely wild.

Norma describes the role of the volunteer. At LifePath Hospice and Palliative Care, volunteers are required to commit to 2 to 4 hours per week with one patient. The volunteer is part of a team that includes a physician who is the medical director of the hospice, the nurse who is the clinical team leader, a counselor, a nurse's aide, and the volunteer coordinator. A chaplain, homemaker, bereavement counselor, and even a beautician may also provide services in a particular case, though they will not attend team meetings. Different levels of service are provided depending on the patient's needs, and not every patient needs every service that is offered. Each clinical team meets once a week to discuss the patients, and not every patient is discussed every week. As a volunteer, I may request to attend the team meeting for my patient, but my volunteer coordinator would be there anyway as my representative. All information is shared, so I will be permitted to read the patient's charts and can ask questions of other team members any time I want to. I will fill out patient notes for every visit that I make. If something urgent comes up, I can call the office and ask to speak to someone immediately.

Norma reassures me, "You should never feel like you're out there on your own—we're always just a phone call away. We also have support meetings for 2 hours every month. You're not required to attend those meetings, but it's a good way to meet other volunteers, to get additional education, and to talk through any issues that come up for you."

I will be required to visit my patient once a week. Through the training, I will learn the guidelines that are intended to ensure I am acting as a member of hospice and not becoming too involved with my patient; for example, I will be encouraged to maintain formality by calling ahead to confirm my appointment and by keeping my home phone number confidential. Norma stresses that it can sometimes be difficult to both care for a patient and maintain the appropriate distance, but that boundaries are very important for the care of both the patient and the volunteer.

"For how long will I see a patient? I mean, how long ..." I trail off, not wanting to say, "until a patient dies."

"The average stay in hospice is 2 months, but that doesn't mean that you'll be visiting a patient for that long. There are many patients who only get referred to hospice when they're actively dying, so you may get to see a patient one time before they die. But there are other patients who are in the program for a couple of years, and some even get better and graduate from the hospice program."

I interject. "They graduate?"

"Yes. It's rare, but it does happen. Sometimes a patient is diagnosed as terminal and then they start receiving hospice services and they get better, so they 'graduate.' The law only allows us to provide services to patients who are dying. Sometimes, a patient will improve because we get their pain under control, or because they start getting social support and contact with the nurse and the volunteer, or they are no longer depressed because they receive counseling."

"Wow. That says a lot about hospice and the care you provide." I feel myself further revising my understanding of hospice. I am surprised and glad to hear of cases where people "get better" and leave the program—even more surprised by the paradox in using a metaphor of academic achievement to describe an event that is *not* expected, where someone *did not* complete the hospice journey.

From the quiet that has descended outside our office I sense that I've probably kept Norma after her business hours. I've been taking notes as we talk but my thoughts are reeling as I contemplate the future. I am both excited and anxious to take the next step.

"So, when can I do the training?"

"I believe our next training will be in February. I'll give you a form to fill out with your name and contact details, and then we can send you an announcement in the mail once the dates have been finalized. You probably won't hear anything until January, but you *will* hear from us."

I'm disappointed. The training won't be for another 2 months. I was hoping to continue the momentum I'd established through this meeting. I hope I don't lose my nerve.

Norma continues, "The good news is, you won't have to go through this interview with me again when you sign up. You can just call and tell us which session you want to attend."

So, this was a kind of screening. I suppose it makes sense that they interview potential volunteers before they enroll in the program, and I'm glad I appear to have passed the test. I wonder what I could have said or done to signal that I wasn't a suitable volunteer. I wonder how many people they turn down, if any. Perhaps because I feel the "interview" was conducted somewhat covertly, I don't feel it would be appropriate to probe Norma about her methods, and besides, it's clearly time for me to go.

Norma asks if I have any more questions or concerns, then walks me out to the foyer.

"I'm so glad to have met you, Elissa," she says, her eyes bright. She reaches out her hand to clasp mine warmly. "I look forward to seeing you at the training."

"I'm glad I came today, too. I'm looking forward to getting started."

"It'll come quickly. In the meantime, good luck and have a great Christmas!"

"Thanks. You too." Then I'm out the glass doors and walking to my car.

As I drive home, I reflect on my conversation with Norma. My thoughts drift backward to memories of my grandmother and then forward to the patients I could meet in the future. Norma made it seem so easy, but I find it difficult to grasp the reality of getting to know someone who is dying. I find it even harder to imagine myself being comfortable, and calm, and supportive in the ways I imagine a hospice volunteer should be. I know that I am carrying the legacy of what transpired with my grandmother. I feel confident that I can handle so many other communication challenges—but not this one.

When I arrive home, I glance at the clock and do a quick mental calculation of the time difference between Tampa and Brisbane.

"She may be home," I think. "I might as well try."

I pick up the phone and dial. The ringing is answered at the other end.

"Hi, Mum," I say. "I just got home. You'll never guess what I did this afternoon."

INTEGRATING THE PRIVATE AND THE PUBLIC

In his book *The Empty Space*, theater director Peter Brook (1968) refers to his creative process as beginning with a "formless hunch" from which he gains inspiration for each choice that he makes, as he literally builds a theatrical production from the ground up. When I moved from Australia to the United States, I moved from an educational background and career in theater to pursue a graduate degree in communication studies—a subject area that did not exist as a single unified discipline within Australia. This enormous life change was driven by a "formless hunch" regarding the connection between relationships and quality of life; I knew that I wanted to have a positive impact on the world through research and teaching about human relationships, but the details of that vision took many years to emerge.

At first, as I undertook my studies of interpersonal and health communication, I eschewed my training in the performing arts in order to adopt the worldview of social science—with its emphasis on measurement, predication, and control—which I accepted as the dominant paradigm of relationship research. When I began the doctoral program in communication at the University of South Florida, however, I was introduced to ethnographic methods and saw the possibility to integrate my social scientific and artistic training. Specifically, the combined perspectives of narrative and autoethnography (Ellis & Bochner, 2000) provided me with a framework for generating evocative research accounts that incorporate both personal experience and theoretical analysis (see the Appendix for an extended discussion of the ethnographic approach used in this study). I realized that, even when working in theater, I had always been a professional observer of human nature and interaction, and had also developed skills of representing life through creative writing. Those skills could now be brought to bear on one of the most important and challenging contexts I could imagine—how to communicate with people as they face the end of their lives. Furthermore, I could take a passion that grew from my personal experience with my grandmother and generate research that could positively impact the lives of others who face similar challenges. With my decision to become a hospice volunteer and write an ethnographic account of my experience, all the pieces began to come together—my communication training, my background in narrative writing, my interest in health and human relationships, and my desire to understand communication at the end of life.

I spent a lot of time thinking about the ethics of my decision to integrate these two goals, because I ran the risk of raising suspicions from both sides. Academic researchers, particularly those of an empiricist bent, might argue that my personal involvement precludes me from bringing a sufficiently objective perspective to my analysis. This criticism is becoming less defensible as the value of subjectivity is more widely demonstrated and articulated within the social sciences. The more difficult criticism I anticipated, and the one that concerned me more, was that I could not be a "true" volunteer if my "real" intention was to conduct research. From the beginning, I made a commitment to be led by my role as a hospice volunteer and to adapt my research process to that commitment—rather than the other way around. The arguments I present here and the results of the research itself—the stories of this book—will permit the reader to judge whether I was successful in my goal of being both a committed volunteer and an effective researcher.

Just as hospice emphasizes care of the "whole person," the "narrative turn" (Bochner, 1994) in ethnographic research has reclaimed the voice of the academic as a whole person (Tompkins, 1996). Many researchers choose to integrate their lives and their work, because it is precisely their personal concerns that drive their interests. Reminding myself of this means that I need not struggle to keep my personal journey separate from my academic writing; each can enrich the other in a text that gives voice to my emotions as well as my thoughts and ideas, and I cannot imagine reaching any understanding of hospice care without my heart's wisdom. I need to be as open as I can about the journey I'm making or, as Tedlock (1991) puts it, "identify the consciousness which has selected and shaped the experiences within the text" (p. 78). I must claim (and will continue to do so throughout the book) theoretical authority as a communication scholar, but my claims will be made more valuable by acknowledging my vulnerability—that I am at a loss for words when faced with the awesome reality of death.

As I began my journey, I again gained comfort from Brook's (1968) description of the "formless hunch," recognizing that sometimes all one has is an intuitive understanding that one is pursuing something important. After I met with Norma, the plan for my project began to emerge and, in this sense, my research was "grounded" in the experience of the field (Glaser & Strauss, 1967). From the beginning, I felt motivated by personal and moral obligations as well as academic ones. In addition to describing pragmatic issues, these and the other methodological asides throughout the book will show how personal experience and intuition have shaped my research and writing processes. Writing is integral to all phases of ethnographic research (Goodall, 2000; Lindlof, 1995). For the ethnographer, writing is both a method of data collection and a process of inquiry (Richardson, 1994) through which the researcher grapples with the challenges of both understanding and representing the experience of the fieldwork. As an ethnographer exploring the role of communication and relationships, my goals are to experience the relationships, events, and emotions of hospice volunteering; to reflect actively on the experience alone and with other volunteers; and to represent those processes evocatively. The ethnographic writing process also helps me to articulate what I am thinking, feeling, and learning along the way, and thus the writing contributes to my personal goal of learning to communicate more humanely when faced with terminal illness and death. As Carey (1992) points out, experience and our accounts of experience are two different things, yet we need accounts in order to share our experiences of the world with one another. My challenge, therefore, is to represent what this experience was like from my perspective, and also to reveal a sense of what it meant to other volunteers, as well as to connect these experiences to communication principles and theories within a broader context of social life. Therefore, it is important to situate my story within the context of the hospice movement and LifePath Hospice as an organization.

DEFINING HOSPICE

The people who first told me about hospice, both health care profession-als and the surviving caregivers of patients, were profoundly grateful and full of praise for hospice workers and the organization. As I listened to their stories, I realized that the word *hospice* refers to a kind of organi-zation and not simply a type of residential facility as it does in Australia. Moreover, the people who had shared their stories of hospice with me came from several regions across the United States, so I concluded that hospice also refers to many different organizations, rather than a single company. Hospice also connotes a philosophy of care as much as it re-fers to a type of health care system. After searching various Web sites to identify hospices in my area, I did not have a clear picture in my mind of what made their approach and services so special. If hospice was suc-cessful in communicating care at the end of life, I needed to understand the organizational context in order to interpret the nature and quality of interactions. I needed to find out more about hospice care in the United States regarding its history and development as both an organization and as a philosophy of end-of-life care.

In their earliest history, hospices are associated with the Christian tradition, although ancient Greek, Roman, and Arabic cultures also es-tablished customs related to the kind treatment of strangers. The word hospice derives from the Latin *hospitium* meaning entertainment, hospi-tality, or lodging (Bennahum, 1996). The first hospices appear to have been founded in the 11th century during the Crusades—specifically, by the Knights Hospitallers—who established places of rest for pilgrims travelling to the Holy Land (Connor, 1998). Further historical origins of hospice are found during the 17th century when St. Vincent de Paul and the Sisters of Charity created homes in France for orphans, the poor, the sick, and the dying (Connor, 1998). The Irish Sisters of Charity founded Our Lady's Hospice in Dublin in 1879, and then St. Joseph's Hospice for the dying poor in London in 1905 (Bennahum, 1996). It was at St. Jo-seph's that Cicely Saunders came to study 50 years later, and developed her theories related to pain management and the needs of dying pa-tients (Connor, 1998). Saunders, who is recognized as the founder of the modern hospice movement, originally trained as a nurse, then as a so-cial worker and physician. She opened St. Christopher's Hospice out-side London in 1967 and established it as "a center of excellence in care of the dying patient" (Connor, 1998, p. 5), which included teaching and research facilities in addition to its hospice services.

The brief history just presented suggests that the development of the hospice movement has been a continuous and unbroken evolution. However, it is important to note that the hospice movement would not exist as it does today in the United States without the significant cultural shift in medical practices that occurred during the 20th century. Particularly after World War II, medical science and its increasingly powerful technologies appropriated the processes of illness and dying (Brand, 1988; Connor, 1998). As Morris (1998) puts it, "It is as if modernist medicine believed that simply by applying enough raw science to the specific causes of illness it could ultimately defeat death" (p. 237). As a result, death became a cultural taboo wherein the person who was dying was "a medical embarrassment" and the bereaved person "a social embarrassment" (Walter, 1994, p. 24). Hospice, therefore, originated as a social movement, which in turn established a model of health care delivery that responded to the inhumanity of the modern way of dying. Walter (1994) saw hospice as part of a "revival" that began in the late 1960s to rehumanize the dying process, to return it to the province of the personal and "to care for and listen to the whole person" (p. 187). As my review of its development demonstrates, the hospice movement continues to grow and respond to changing sociopolitical conditions.

Although Cicely Saunders's work with hospice in England grew directly from existing religious charities, the development of the hospice movement in the United States was somewhat different. In 1963, Saunders was invited to speak at the Yale University School of Medicine, where she met Florence Wald, dean of the graduate school of nursing. In 1974, after studying with Saunders at St. Christopher's, Wald opened the home care component of Connecticut Hospice Inc., which was the first hospice in the United States (Friedrich, 1999). Seale (1998) convincingly argued that the U.S. interest in hospice was fueled simultaneously by the success of numerous publications that appeared between 1965 and 1969, critiquing modern medicine's approach to dying. Among these publications, Seale noted Glaser and Strauss's *Awareness of Dying* (1965) and *Time for Dying* (1968), and Kübler-Ross's *On Death and Dying* (1969). Residential hospices and inpatient units constitute one facet of end-of-life care; however, from these early days on, the U.S. hospice movement focused on home care rather than inpatient services (Bennahum, 1996; Connor, 1998; Miller, Mor, Gage, & Coppola, 2000). Hospice is now well established as an attractive alternative to the dehumanization associated with dying in the modern medical system (Seale, 1998).

The hospice movement grew rapidly. The National Hospice and Palliative Care Organization (NHPCO)—originally the National Hospice Organization—was founded in 1978, and the first national directory published that year listed 1,200 hospices (Connor, 1998). The purpose of the NHPCO was "to establish guidelines for operational issues necessary to develop hospice programs" (Bennahum, 1996, p. 6), as well as to educate the public and advocate for the hospice philosophy of care for the dying (Miller et al., 2000). Since the founding of the NHPCO, two important professional developments have occurred. In 1993, the NHPCO published its *Standards of a Hospice Program of Care* as a comprehensive set of norms representing excellence in hospice practice, and in 1995 the Joint Commission for Accreditation of Health Care Organizations offered accreditation to hospices under the home health accreditation program (Connor, 1998, p. 99). There are now numerous national organizations that attempt to improve quality of care in the hospice industry. They include National Association for Home Care, Hospice Association of America, Foundation for Hospice and Home Care, Hospice Education Institute, Children's Hospice International, and National Institute for Jewish Hospice. The NHPCO also has state-affiliated organizations that serve similar functions (Hayslip & Leon, 1992). These various professional organizations represent multiple levels of supervision that affect the daily running of a hospice program in the United States, but systems of financial reimbursement are an even more pervasive force that influences the life of hospice.

In 1982, hospice was added as a Medicare benefit and Medicare began to pay for services the following year. Although hospice initially resisted both Medicare and accreditation structures as antithetical to the charitable philosophy of hospice (Connor, 1998), by 1998, 80% of hospices participated in Medicare reimbursement (Moore, 1998). This change was to have a lasting impact on the structure and services of hospice in the United States; it ensured ongoing financial support for hospice across the country and also added a new level of bureaucracy to the system. Regarding Medicare, one hospice researcher states "It converts hospice to much more of a business .... On the other hand, it made hospice available to a whole lot of people that were never going to get it on a volunteer basis" (Moore, 1998, p. 39). Figures from the official NHPCO Web site illustrate the growth of hospice since the introduction of the Medicare benefit. During 1985, the first census year, 158,000 people were enrolled in 1,545 hospice programs; in 2002, the latest census year, 885,000 people were served by over 3,200 hospices (NHPCO, n.d.). Perhaps more significant are statistics provided by the NHPCO, which state that compared to all Americans who died in 2003, patients in hospice care were twice as likely to die at home and 80% less likely to die in a hospital. Of the estimated 1.7 million people over the age of 65 who died in 1996 in the U.S., almost 18% were enrolled in Medicare's hospice benefit, which paid for 77% of all hospice care in the United States that year (Miller et al., 2000). In 2003, 94.7% of all hospices were Medicare certified (NHPCO, n.d).

Along with the Medicare benefit came increased surveillance by the Health Care Finance Administration. In 1993, some hospices in Puerto Rico were reported to be abusing Medicare funding, which led to Operation Restore Trust (Moore, 1998). In 1995, as a direct result of this investigation, the first guidelines for determining prognosis in noncancer patients were published by the NHPCO. These guidelines were designed to standardize the admission criteria for noncancer patients under Medicare but, as borne out by the stories in this book, establishing accurate prognoses for these patients remains notoriously difficult (Miller, et al., 2000). Although the Medicare benefit theoretically allows an unlimited stay, to be admitted to hospice, a physician must assess a patient's life expectancy to be 6 months or less. Patients are then periodically reassessed, may be discharged from hospice (or "graduate"), and can be readmitted when, once again, they fit the guidelines. Christakis and Iwashyna's study (cited in Miller et al., 2000, p. 196) suggested that the recent rise in late referrals to hospice is a direct consequence of these guidelines and increased scrutiny by the offices of the Inspector General and the Health Care Finance Administration. Late referral greatly reduces the impact that a hospice program can have on quality of life, particularly if patients are admitted only days or hours before their death. The same agencies that contributed to the growth of the hospice movement by financially supporting hospice care may also undermine its effectiveness by inappropriately restricting access (Shapiro, 1997). One hospice attempted to circumvent the problems associated with the 6-month Medicare rule. With the help of a grant from the Robert Wood Johnson Foundation, Hospice of the Valley in Phoenix developed and implemented a pilot program that provided palliative care for chronically ill patients who were still seeking curative treatment prior to admission to hospice (Hickey, 1999; Lockhart, Volk-Craft, Hamilton, Aiken, & Williams, 2003). As the average age of the population continues to increase, the human costs of the current Medicare bureaucracy may well incite widespread revision of hospice goals and services, to encompass a broader understanding of end-of-life issues and a more inclusive definition of the appropriate hospice patient.

As I consider the history of the hospice movement and its growth in the United States, the number and variety of stakeholders I have encountered surprise me. What began in 1974 as a small, home care organization has burgeoned into a vast and complex system that reaches from the level of federal government reimbursement and professional supervision and accreditation to the level of individual citizens who seek an alternate experience of dying. Although my primary research interest is in understanding the human interaction between hospice volunteers and patients at the end of life, I wonder how the historical and institutional context of hospice affects those interactions. The hospice literature rarely mentions the role of the volunteer in relation to patient care, except to say that volunteers are an essential characteristic of a hospice program (Connor, 1998). My work as a volunteer may be largely invisible in the hospice story as told from the perspective of policy makers and financial stakeholders, but this does not mean that I am outside or beyond the reach of the bureaucracy they constitute.

The organizational context of my study, LifePath Hospice and Palliative Care (hereafter called LifePath Hospice) was established in 1983 and is now one of the largest hospices in the United States. In terms of its structure, purpose, and patient population, LifePath Hospice represents a typical example of hospice organizations in the United States (see the Appendix). As noted earlier in this chapter, hospice care in the United States is largely focused on home care rather than inpatient services (Bennahum, 1996; Connor, 1998). In addition to caring for patients in their own homes, LifePath Hospice provides care to residents in nursing homes, assisted living facilities, and the residential Hospice House, which opened in 2001. Conforming to hospice philosophies and accepted practices, LifePath Hospice employs an interdisciplinary approach to care that includes a medical director, nurses, social workers, a chaplain, home health aids, therapists, and bereavement counselors. As a not-for-profit organization receiving Medicare funds, LifePath Hospice is also supported by hundreds of volunteers assigned to several kinds of duties including home care, nursing home care, administrative duties such as office work and fundraising, work with children, bereavement counseling, and community education.

Although I am interested in studying the interaction between hospice volunteers and patients, the impact of hospice history, organizational culture, and structure on that interaction should not be underestimated. The diagnosis and prognosis of a hospice patient, the timing of a patient's referral and admission to hospice, the complicated reimbursement systems that can interfere with or determine how pain is managed—all these factors can impact the relationship between the volunteer and the patient. As an interpersonal communication scholar who conducted an ethnographic study, I have the benefit of being able to focus on individual-level interactions while recognizing the impact of context on those interactions. The interactions between volunteers and patients are meaningful because they are unique and, at the same time, the relationships between volunteers and patients are framed by the culture of the hospice organization that defines the role of the volunteer in a particular way. Also, the historical developments that led to the stigmatization of dying in our culture continue to affect our attitudes and expectations about the end of life. The characteristics of volunteer–patient interaction that interest me as a communication researcher—for example, the characteristics of conversation and disclosure, the negotiation of power and control, and the role of gestures and silence in developing relationships—are both unique expressions and also indicative of patterns that occur within specific cultural and organizational contexts. Ethnographic narrative writing permits me to move between these different frames, focusing in on the details of an interaction or story then stepping back to interpret the meaning of the interaction in terms of what it says about communication and relationships at the end of life.

By observing, recording, analyzing and representing the details of lived experience in hospice, I draw attention to aspects and qualities of interactions that may be overlooked or taken for granted in the course of providing hospice care; and yet, from a relational perspective (Rogers & Escudero, 2004), these interactions constitute the essence of care that hospice provides. Being within a caring relationship and being able to reflect on it with the perspective of a communication scholar, I hope to articulate lessons and insights from the experience that will contribute to the understanding of those who work in hospice, those who volunteer or who want to volunteer, and those who may need to engage the services of hospice for themselves or for a loved one.

As I describe in the next chapter, my first step toward gaining a practical understanding and experience of hospice care was to undertake 20 hours of volunteer training at LifePath Hospice. My role as a volunteer was foundational to this study, because I began from an acknowledged position of naiveté, with the hope that I would learn through experience and take readers with me on the journey. In addition to preparing me to do the work of a volunteer, the training program provided me with a structured period of socialization into the culture of hospice through which I was able to gain an understanding of "what it's like around here" by reflecting on and questioning the taken-for-granted aspects of the training.

ANTICIPATION

As Norma predicted, 2 months passed before I heard from LifePath Hospice about the training. I wondered if this was another test of my commitment and suitability for the program. The night before the first session, I am nervous and excited, trying to imagine what tomorrow will bring. The training I attended as a hospital volunteer focused on infection control, emergency procedures, safety, and patient confidentiality laws. Probably some of the same information will be covered tomorrow, but there is much more I need to know if I hope to be comfortable talking to people about dying. As a hospital volunteer, I interacted with patients only intermittently as I attended to my assigned duties of fetching water and blankets, transporting patients, collecting records, and emptying urinals. When I talked with patients and was able to comfort them I felt more useful and needed than at any other time, but those moments were special partly because they were outside the norm. In hospice, my primary duty will be to engage in close, personal interactions with patients. How will I learn to *make* this happen when it is not simply incidental?

I imagine the scene. "Hi, my name is Elissa Foster and, now that you're dying, hospice has sent me to be your friend."

I wince.

My thoughts turn to tomorrow's training session, and I wonder who else will be there.

2

Volunteer Training

ARRIVING

I pull into the parking lot at 8.50 a.m., with 10 minutes to spare. As I walk toward the front door, I notice two other women approaching the entrance. The first woman greets me, and from her welcoming and relaxed demeanor, I surmise that she is one of the trainers. I ask for directions and she points me through the same doors I entered back in December. I hear the second woman behind me as I walk through the foyer. When I turn to hold the door for her, I notice that she's young, probably in her early 20s.

"Is it down this way?" the young woman asks.

"Yes," I reply. "You're here for the training, obviously. So am I."

"Yes. Hi, I'm Sarah," she says.

"Elissa," I hold out my hand. "Good to meet you."

We reach the end of the corridor and enter a small room with glass walls where we fill out nametags and add our names to a list of 11 people already signed in. Beyond this room is a larger one set up with a long narrow table stretching across the length of the room with a thick, three-ring binder in front of every seat. Behind the table is a supply of juice, coffee, fruit, muffins, and Danish pastries. The word *abundance* comes to mind; this room makes me feel that the trainers have considered our needs and they will take care of us. In the midst of the uncertainty, I relax. I walk to the far side of the table, settle into a chair and pull out my notepad and pen—a willing and compliant student. The familiar actions calm my nerves, and I wonder what we will talk about for 9 hours today.

The two hospice trainers, Patrice and Karen, are organized, calm, friendly, and professional. They hand us an agenda for the series of three training sessions, a folder for our handouts, and then direct our attention to the 160-page manual in our three-ring binder, which covers all areas of the training. According to the agenda, we will complete our communication training first, followed by patient care skills, and then family dynamics. The following week we will cover spiritual care, signs and symptoms of dying, boundaries, grief, and a session called Volunteer Connection. Our graduation will be held the last Monday night of the training. As I consider the topics and note the size of the manual, I am both reassured and intimidated—reassured that the trainers have anticipated how much we need to learn, and intimidated by the prospect of having to absorb so much in two 9-hour sessions. I wonder if we will spend much time talking among ourselves, and whether I will get to know anyone.

I scan the room and count 14 participants including myself. My mind switches to researcher mode and I gauge the diversity; as far as I can tell, we range in age between 20 and 50. There are 4 men and 10 women: three are African American, two are Latino, and nine are White. When we introduce ourselves around the table, I learn more about the group. For instance, four of us were born outside the United States or have family members overseas; seven of us are students, including five undergraduate and two doctoral students; one is a disabled Vietnam veteran; one is a psychologist in private practice; and one is an attorney. I listen carefully to everyone's stories about why he or she wants to volunteer. Some, like me, have past experiences of losing someone close to them; I speculate about the stories that we are not sharing.

COMMUNICATION IN HOSPICE

During our communication training, Patrice, the primary trainer, advises us to listen and not judge or impose our values onto patients and their families, even when it comes to evidence of racism, sexism, or homophobia. When she asks us to consider whose needs are being met when we impose our values onto the hospice patient and family, I perceive a dilemma. Norma suggested that volunteers should be honest about what makes us uncomfortable so that we don't put our patients and ourselves in an awkward situation. But Patrice seems to suggest that it is selfish not to look past something like racism. I am confused about how to negotiate these contradictory mandates to consider the needs and the perspective of the patient, and simultaneously honor my own need to feel safe and comfortable. It's also hard to imagine these complex negotiations in the hypothetical, without an actual relationship within which to judge the soundness of this advice. Nevertheless, the guidelines that Patrice is offering emphasize a general principle of centering on the needs of the patients and adapting our communication to their worldview and preferences.

Patrice's advice suggests that adapting to our patients is an essential characteristic of our communication as volunteers. This adaptation goes beyond simply accepting or overlooking a patient's or family's values or beliefs if they differ from our own. I am reminded of one of Walter's (1994) observations about hospice as a philosophy and system of care, particularly the idea of adapting to the needs of individual patients and families. Walter (1994) asks a series of questions that highlight the practical challenges of enacting the principle of individualized care:

> How, in practice, does the practitioner listen to each and every individual passing through a palliative care unit, funeral parlor, or bereavement agency? .... Can *systems* be developed for something so personal? Can death be tailored according to personal preference? (Walter, 1994, p. 87)

It is a primary goal of hospice to treat each person as an individual and to respect the feelings, beliefs, and wishes of the dying person. Cicely Saunders, founder of the modern hospice movement, envisioned the communication between hospice workers and families as one of dialogue, an explicitly "I and Thou" relationship (Bradshaw, 1996) as described by the philosopher Martin Buber (1970; 1988). Ideally, this relationship is one in which the particular values, personalities, or life circumstances of the hospice workers (including volunteers) or patients do not present a barrier to the delivery of holistic care (Bradshaw, 1996). Even as I recognize the relevance of dialogue as a principle for volunteers, I recall that Buber himself argued in his dialogue with Carl Rogers (Anderson & Cissna, 1997) that true dialogue is limited within an unequal "helping" relationship, such as the volunteer– patient relationship, and tends to be momentary when it does occur.

Our ability to achieve the ideals of dialogue are both facilitated and complicated by the practice of multidisciplinary teamwork in hospice. Seale (1998) identified the emergence of multidisciplinary health care teams as part of a larger movement toward patient-centered medicine and away from anatomo-clinical medicine, which had made the voice of the patient less relevant. The concept of teams in health care delivery both recognizes the worth of various specialties and recasts the "relations between members of the formal health care team and 'clients' or informal members of the team" (Seale, 1998, p. 97). The volunteer role is the least defined of all the hospice team member roles, and shares similar characteristics with what Seale (1998) called the *informal* members of the team. Although Seale used this term to refer to the patient and family, their roles are informal because they do not have to answer to hospice and they have a great deal of flexibility regarding the way they choose to live and to respond to dying. Similarly, there are just as many variations and manifestations of the volunteer role as there are ways to be a caregiver or a patient, which suggests that the volunteer is also an informal role within the hospice team. As a member of the team, I am encouraged to act autonomously and to improvise as I discover what is required of my role as a volunteer. Ideally, this freedom allows all team members to respond directly to a patient's needs without worrying whether or not it is part of their assigned jobs. However, as I recall from my experiences working in theater, improvisation demands a high degree of skill, familiarity with the context and the role one is playing, and enough confidence to surrender to the moment (Eisenberg, 1990). Walter's (1994) critique of hospice suggests that practitioners and families (and, no doubt, volunteers) sometimes find it challenging to negotiate the ambiguity of such open guidelines.

In our session with Patrice, we also discuss listening as a crucial communication skill for hospice workers because it retains focus on the patient and family (Butler, Burt, Foley, Morris, & Morrison, 1996; Connor, 1998; Walter, 1996). I recall that in one study, "active listening" was ranked as the most frequently implemented nursing intervention used to "enhance and support the spirituality of clients and their families" (Sellers & Haag, 1998, pp. 347–348). I was intrigued to see listening described as an "intervention," because it suggested a nondirective behavior intended to support the patient but for a specific and intentional outcome. Again, I was reminded of Walter's (1996) critique as he provocatively described what may be a fundamental tension in the hospice movement:

> On the one hand, they are committed to letting patients live as they wish until they die. On the other hand, hospices have a very clear idea of "the good death" .... These are the two classic strands that together make a revival: a late-modern/ neo-traditional attempt to promote a particular idea of healthy dying, and a postmodern enabling of individuals to do it their own way. (p. 89)

Although Walter's comments are directed toward hospice as a philosophy and social movement, I can see how this tension—between encouraging the patient's autonomy and remaining nondirective while advocating a "good death"— must also affect the day-to-day relationships and communication between hospice workers and patients. As I listen to the discussion and think about my role as a volunteer, I anticipate that I will need to negotiate between the directives of the organization, my patient's wishes, and my own values.

During this first day of training, I experience many moments of thinking that I understand the information, but without a frame of reference for how to put it into practice. For example, Patrice advises us to "be a nonanxious presence" and "be who we are"; I understand the idea but question my ability to achieve it when I am with a patient. Having learned through years of schooling to trust my intellect, I realize that it may not help me at all in this endeavor; rather, I will have to learn through experience. At the end of the day, after sessions on patient care and family dynamics, we discuss our fears about volunteering and I learn that others feel the same way that I do. Two of the other volunteers reflect my feelings particularly well. Henry, a quiet man in his mid-40s, says he fears saying the wrong thing or not knowing what to say at all. Ela, a pre-med student in her early 20s, says that she fears being overwhelmed by the families' emotions when their loved one is dying. We want to respond in helpful and positive ways to our prospective patients and their families, and yet we still feel ill-equipped, tongue-tied, and anxious. In response to some of these fears, Patrice restates two ideas from today's session. She says, "We are not change agents. We are there to bear witness, to support, and to comfort." It all makes sense—in theory.

SECOND DAY OF TRAINING

When I arrive at the LifePath offices I immediately sense that everyone feels more comfortable with each other and with the environment. I take the same seat and begin a conversation with two of my neighbors at the table: Chris, an African American social work student, and Emilia, a graphic designer from Brazil. Patrice, our trainer, is already here. As the chatter in the room dies down a little, my attention is drawn to her. Patrice is talking about hospice organizational structure, reimbursement for hospice services, and the role of the volunteers. The training has not officially started for the day, but someone has asked Patrice about how volunteers fit into the larger organization. At the hospital, I often felt like I was "free labor" and not an important contributor to the work of the hospital. Here, I already feel that hospice values my role and my contribution. I am not just free labor; I am an essential component of what distinguishes hospice from other types of end-of-life care.

Our second day of training officially begins when Karen, a trainer, introduces a videotape of an episode from *Nightline*, which compiles three interviews with Morrie Schwartz, whose last days are recounted in Mitch Albom's (1997) bestseller *Tuesdays with Morrie*. The *Nightline* interviews were conducted over 6 months in 1995, leading up to the last days of Morrie's life (Morris, 1995). I watch and listen intently to what Morrie says about his approaching death. Two themes recur throughout: Morrie's definition of what makes his life worth living, and his acceptance of the changes in his body and the lessons being revealed to him through the process of dying.

The other volunteers also study the screen; some are teary-eyed. Although Karen didn't introduce the video in this way, Morrie seems to be presented as an "ideal" hospice patient—articulate and willing to express his feelings and thoughts about dying. I believe I will know how to interact with a patient like Morrie; at the same time, I doubt that I will meet someone who is as open and self-reflexive as he is. I worry that, in this context, he represents a stereotype of "a dying person" that we may internalize, only to be surprised when we meet our "real" patients.

I don't know how I would establish a relationship with a patient who cannot speak. I also feel unprepared to engage in the kinds of conversations about death and dying depicted on the *Nightline* video, unless it is with someone who is as articulate as Morrie. Discourse plays a central role in hospice, especially to the concept of "the good death."

THE ROLE OF "TALK" IN HOSPICE

For communication scholars, the term *discourse* can imply two distinct focal points of study. For those who study communication at a cultural level, discourse refers to a system of language within a given context, as in, medical discourse, political discourse, or feminist discourse. Discourse in this sense reflects the work of philosopher Michel Foucault, who identified it as systems of symbols or language (spoken or written, mediated or unmediated) that are internally consistent, belong to identifiable groups or movements, express values and orientations, and are held to be normative or persuasive (Baglia, 2005; Coupland & Gwynn, 2003). The discourse that we adopt can affect what we believe and how we feel about the phenomena to which it refers. An important contribution that hospice has made as a social movement is the construction of a revised discourse related to death and dying. So far in the training, I had already noticed some of the hospice terminology used by the trainers such as the *good death, hospice patient, imminent separation,* and *actively dying*. According to a social constructionist perspective, language creates our reality (Berger & Luckmann, 1967; Gergen, 1994), and from this perspective, language is vital to hospice as a revivalist movement that hopes to change our social understanding of death and treatment of people who are dying.

In its second meaning, discourse can also refer to conversational exchange, wherein language is the medium of social interaction between individuals. This second usage is closely related to the first, because as language is exchanged through conversation or *talk*, the content of that talk—the language that is available to express the meanings of the speakers—is constrained by the dominant cultural discourse. Even whether or not we are expected to talk about certain things—such as death and dying—is affected by discursive conventions. Seale (1998) suggests that discourse in this second sense is also central to hospice philosophy and care, because hospice relies on language as an essential component of the meaningful death, particularly in the patient's ability to articulate his or her thoughts and emotions as death approaches. However, Seale (1998) warns that hospice practitioners should be careful not to focus too much attention on conversational discourse or "talk" in the provision of care, because it is easy to overlook the physical manifestation of death as a site of meaning, particularly for the person who is dying.

Our bodies make us undeniably mortal and it is our symbolic constructions—our words—that ward off our sense of mortality and extend us toward eternity (Becker, 1997). Because language has the power to disassociate us from our mortality—our bodies—it has become, ironically, the power we turn to at the hour of our death. As a communication scholar, I am provoked and intrigued by Walter's (1994) and Seale's (1998) critiques of the centrality of talk in the "revivalist" practices of hospice. In particular, Seale (1998) warns of a potential methodological danger associated with our reliance on talk. He suggests that despite the intention of researchers who use qualitative interviewing and narrative inquiry to empower the voice of the research participant, these methods almost inevitably disembody the subject, "due to the emphasis on symbolic manipulation through talk" (p. 28). Thus, even as we use interviews to try to understand the experiences of people who are dying and their caregivers, we run the risk of overlooking the impact of bodily experience because we focus on thoughts and words; we also risk privileging cognitive responses rather than instinctive or emotional responses.

As I watch the video of Morrie Schwartz, I hear him describe his body's physical disintegration from the effects of ALS (Lou Gehrig's Disease). But rather than feeling emotionally overwhelmed by his graphic descriptions, I hear his words and feel cognitively comforted because he is "still there," he is "still able to communicate," and he is "still human" because he can share his internal life with the interviewer and with us, the audience. In doing so, I note that I am falling into a cultural habit of my Western upbringing by equating Morrie's mind with his "true self," as though his body is merely a container that is deteriorating as the real Morrie goes on unchanged. I begin to consider the aspects of his experience that are inexpressible. As I remember the critiques I have read, I am prompted to examine my assumptions and attitudes about hospice patients who cannot, for whatever reason, express themselves in words.

PHYSICAL DEATH IN HOSPICE

In the second half of today's training session, we turn to the difficult subject of signs and symptoms at the end of life, led by one of the hospice nurses, Carson Riley.

Carson begins, "Hospice takes what is called a 'holistic' approach to the care of the dying. So far, you've discussed communication, emotions, and your role as volunteers who provide support for patients and their families. I'm here to describe the physical aspects, so you can better understand what happens to the body when your patient is actively dying. Although time of death is very difficult to predict, there are changes that tell us when a patient is approaching death and likely to die in the coming hours or days."

Carson tells us that, first, the blood goes toward the major organs of the body and we will be able to observe a change in the skin's temperature; fever is common in the dehydrated patient, but the patient's skin can also become cooler. The color of a patient's skin may also change. As patients lose their ability to control their bladder and bowel toward the end of life, hospice may elect to put in a Foley catheter for urination, which also helps the caregivers because they don't have to worry about keeping the patients dry or changing the bedding.

"As death approaches," Carson says, "the patient will tend to sleep more; this is normal. One thing that you may want to remember is that hearing is the last thing to go, so it is a good idea to keep speaking to your patients so they know someone is there with them." Carson describes how there can be a certain amount of disorientation and confusion, which is caused by a buildup of ammonia in the bloodstream as the body shuts down. We may also observe behaviors that seem strange but are not necessarily disorientation; for example, patients may talk about people who have died or see people in the room who aren't there. "If this happens," Carson instructs, "feel free to ask the patient who or what they are seeing and just go with what they say."

In their book *Final Gifts*, hospice nurses Maggie Callanan and Patricia Kelley (1992) documented dozens of cases in which patients experience what the authors called Nearing Death Awareness. When Carson mentions this phenomenon of seeing other people in the room, I recall these intriguing stories. The central message of the book is that people who are dying will often communicate in ways that are unfamiliar to us, often in metaphors related to traveling or moving, and we must listen for clues. I turn my attention back to Carson's presentation.

Carson continues with a discussion of one of the more distressing symptoms of dying, often called the "death rattle," which is a build-up of mucus at the back of the throat. As the patient breathes, the mucus moves causing the rattle sounds. If the patient is receiving morphine, there can also be an excess of saliva, but hospice never uses a suction machine to clear the throat because it causes more mucus. Instead, Carson instructs us on how to use sponges to swab the patient's mouth. She holds up a short, plastic stick with a small sponge attached to the end of it. We learn that these sticks can also help if the patient can no longer swallow to drink but their mouth is dry. Although the rattling may sound bad, as if the patient is suffocating, Carson assures us that they are not in distress. If the patient were really air hungry, we would see more physical struggle, but when it is a death rattle, the patients are unresponsive. The sound is most distressing for those who don't know how to interpret it.

"It is also normal for the patient's intake of food and drink to decrease, and this can be particularly distressing for the family," Carson explains. "But if the body is starting to shut down, it can be beneficial for the patient to be somewhat dehydrated, otherwise fluids can build up in the lungs and cause extra respiratory distress. The position we take on artificial hydration and feeding through intravenous fluids or tube feedings is that it is much harder to make the decision to stop those measures than it is to decide not to start."

I think of the protracted battle over Terry Shiavo's life and death at a hospice in Pinellas, Florida, not far from where we are attending this training. Since 1990, Terry Schiavo had been in a persistent vegetative state, kept alive through medical intervention despite her husband's successful—yet contested—court hearings to allow her to die (Hook & Mueller, 2005; Perry, Churchill, & Kirschner, 2005). Although I felt compassion for Terry's parents, who fought to preserve Terry's life in any form, I think about how different Terry's story would have been if her family had decided not to have a feeding tube inserted in the first place.

Tom, one of the trainees, asks how easy is it to predict when a patient is going to die.

Carson responds, "Each case is so different that it can be quite difficult to predict the time of death, although family members do expect hospice to give them more certainty than we really can." She tells the story of an end-stage patient with Chronic, Obstructive Pulmonary Disease (COPD) who had an active day with her family, and a visit from the hospice nurse.

Then, she died that night. The family was upset because they felt the nurse should have warned them. She also tells us that, at other times, a patient may continue to live long after it first appears that death is imminent. Some patients can live 2 to 3 weeks with no food intake at all; sometimes patients will also hold on for a special date or for a relative to visit from out of town.

Carson concludes, "So, hospice will never say, 'This is when your loved one is going to pass,' because we can't ever know for sure. What we *will* do is try to educate the family about what to expect, to prepare them, and to provide as much support as they need toward the end. Sometimes there's a mismatch between the ability of the family member to be there at the end, and the needs or desires of the patient and we try to mediate by providing support services. The worst thing is when caregivers panic at the prospect of someone dying in their house; they call 9-1-1 and the patient gets taken to the hospital. That happens more than you would imagine."

Another trainee, Stephanie, asks, "Are all hospice deaths really free of pain?"

"That's certainly a goal," Carson replies, "but the truth is that we are unable to fully control the pain of 15 to 20% of our patients. The reason for that is *not* that we don't have the medications available or we don't know how to control the pain, it's that the primary care doctor is unwilling to write orders for the quantity of medication that is required."

I have heard about problems related to medication at the end of life. There appear to be two camps, with hospice on one side and primary care doctors and hospitals on the other. The hospice approach is to prescribe whatever quantity of narcotic is necessary to control pain so that patients are able to focus on other things that contribute to their quality of life. Sometimes the narcotic is used to help patients rest peacefully once they have reached a point of actively dying. The traditional biomedical practice is to avoid over prescribing narcotics so that the patients do not spend their last days heavily sedated or become addicted. To me, concern about addiction makes no sense when a person has only a few days to live. It seems to me that it is a misguided sense of morality that has such damaging consequences for people who are dying.

Next to me, Chris raises his hand and asks, "How do we, the volunteers, come away from attending a death, then go about doing our daily business?"

It is a difficult question, but one that I think has been on our minds. Patrice tells us that counseling is available through hospice if we need it, and Carson observes that volunteers naturally get close to their patients, but neither of them really addresses Chris's question. Perhaps this is yet another aspect of volunteering that they can't teach in the training.

By the time the day ends at 5 p.m., I am exhausted. I have 16 pages of notes and the recognition that I will never remember everything. I can hardly believe the training is essentially over now and I could be assigned a patient within a few days.

GRADUATION

On the Monday evening after our second training session, we all gather once more at the LifePath Hospice offices to participate in our graduation ceremony. The evening begins when the head of the volunteer department, Lynne O'Connell, speaks to us about "taking the stuff from the training book and putting it into your heart," meaning that we should internalize the information rather than attempt to go "by the book." I immediately think that she must know what's on my mind— that I don't know enough to begin visiting a patient. I have visions of hauling out my handbook mid-visit to look up strategies to help me.

Three volunteers have come to share their stories with us. We are surprised to learn that one of the speakers, Stephanie, is from our training group and was asked to visit a patient and come back to reassure us about the first visit.

Stephanie begins, "I visited my first patient in a nursing home; she is a young woman, in her 30s, and she has AIDS. First I felt a little nervous about how she would perceive me, but then I thought 'To heck with it. If she likes me, she likes me. If she doesn't, she doesn't, and she can always get another hospice volunteer.

"But actually, I didn't have a problem. She's very open, very talkative. She is new to the program so we didn't have the psychological report back—I didn't know anything about her. One bad moment was when I saw these pictures of this cute little girl. I said, 'What a cute little girl! Who is she?' And she said, 'Oh, that's my daughter.' And I said, 'Well, she's absolutely adorable! How old is she?' And she said, 'Well, she was 5 then. She died.'

"I felt like I put my foot in my mouth. So, I said, 'I'm sorry to hear about that. She's an absolutely beautiful girl.' And she said, 'Well, she ended up having AIDS.' So, evidently she passed it through when she had the child and that's how she found out she had it. So, I was caught off guard, but I kept on going. She didn't break down and cry or anything. We just talked. She's got a lot of people who come to see her, but I think she wanted someone she could talk separately with, you know, a friend."

Chris asks, "What was the nursing home like?"

Stephanie shakes her head a little, then says, "I did tell Patrice that if my mother hadn't worked at a nursing home and my father hadn't been in the hospital so much, I probably wouldn't have gone there because it was wild, very chaotic—a lot of people in wheelchairs always coming up to talk, touch you, and you don't know what to say or do. You don't want to be rude or anything—but when you're going to see a patient you want to focus on them and other people want your attention, too. It's hard to say, 'I'm just here for them.'"

Hannah, another of the trainees, asks, "Did you know that she had AIDS before you went to visit her?"

"Yes," Stephanie responds, "I was told that she was diagnosed with AIDS and asked if that was a problem for me. I said, 'No.' In fact, my patient came right out and asked me if I knew what she had. And I said, 'Yes, I do.' Then she started educating me. I said, 'Great. I don't know anything about it. I'm not a nurse or anything like that so I really don't know.' She was very open and told me what she knew. She just is real nice. Some people because of their condition have a pissed-off attitude. She's just filled with love and she's very well-liked at the nursing home."

After the question and answer period for the panel of speakers, our graduation ceremony begins. The commissioning ceremony is quite moving, particularly when Carla, one of the guest speakers, plays "Amazing Grace"for us. The whole event has a feeling of ritual and solemnity that helps me to feel I have accomplished something significant, and that I am, despite my fears, ready to begin volunteering. We are each awarded a certificate and provided with a collection of supplies including a LifePath Hospice tee shirt. Carla says if we need a ride or a favor from a stranger, we should wear the hospice tee shirt because hospice has helped so many people that they will often go out of their way to help us if they know we are volunteers. Carla shares this information in a fun and lighthearted way, and yet her off-hand comment conveys something significant about our changed status. We were now insiders, a part of hospice.

REFLECTIONS: HOSPICE VOLUNTEER TRAINING

Lynne O'Connell's advice to take the lessons of the training and "put them into our hearts" was a metaphor that emphasized the volunteers' internalization of both hospice guidelines and values. In the ritual, the music, and the language of the graduation ceremony, I also perceived the training to be a process of acculturation or conversion, which resonated with hospice's religious origins. As I described in the first chapter, the services now performed by hospice were historically the province of religious organizations, and even today church-run hospices care for 5 to 10% of hospice patients in the United States (Moore, 1998). Although Saunders established the modern hospice movement under an inclusive and universal definition of spirituality, there are ways in which religion remains evident in norms or "constitutive rules" (Giddens, 1984), which tell volunteers how they are expected to perform, particularly in terms of their commitment to the work. For example, in one article, a hospice manager says of her organization's rigorous volunteer training, "If it's not in the marrow of their soul, they don't stay" (Moore, 1998, p. 41). This statement suggests that hospice work is a vocation, rather than simply a job or even a hobby.

It was clear to me by the end of the training that belief in the hospice philosophy is foundational to the activities performed by members of hospice as an organization (Johanson & Johanson, 1996). As we became socialized or acculturated into hospice, stories of past successes help us to internalize the beliefs of the hospice vision, so that it became "subjectively meaningful" to us (Berger & Luckmann, 1967, p. 129). Thus, the philosophical underpinnings of hospice generate what Berger and Luckmann (1967) call habitualization, a "specialization of activity that ... reliev[es] the accumulation of tensions that result from undirected drives" (p. 53). Throughout our training, the volunteers' various expressions of commitment indicated a rational acceptance and adoption of the hospice philosophy, but also the presence of an emotional connection to the work. Barbalet (1998) argues that emotions exist on a continuum with rationality, and help to direct our sense of purpose. For us to proceed in the face of our anxiety, and to continue volunteering once we encounter challenges, our emotions must motivate us and provide our sense of purpose. Inspirational stories of hospice successes project us into the future with faith that the hospice way is "the right way" and that we will be able to handle whatever lies ahead.

Barbalet (1998) also sheds light on the question of what motivates individuals to engage in hospice volunteering. He describes the self-interest theory of rationality, noting that it limits rational action to "that which serves the actor's self-interest" (p. 40). However, the self-interest theory does not adequately account for the motives of people who are committed to socially responsive behavior—such as volunteering for hospice—that may compromise opportunities for other material goals to be reached. Responding to this weakness in the self-interest theory, Barbalet (1998) turns to the writing of Robert Frank, who suggests a qualification to the theory rather than an outright rejection of it:

> The narrowly conceived self-interest theory of rationality defines the self-interested actor from a limited and individualistic perspective. Taking into account an actor's emotional commitments broadens the scope of their opportunities and satisfactions, and therefore redefines the goals or purposes which must be satisfied if an actor's self-interest is to be better understood and more fully realized. (pp. 40–41)

From Frank's perspective, our motivation to volunteer for hospice cannot be understood simply in terms of rational self-interest as distinct from irrational (or emotional) altruism. Rather, our act of visiting with hospice patients demonstrates a commitment to a greater social good, and also contributes to the attainment of individual or self-interested goals.

The speakers at our graduation echoed a sentiment that was expressed throughout the training—that we would get more out of volunteering than the patients would. A similar sentiment expressed by

experienced hospice volunteers was that "volunteering is so rewarding," yet they did not articulate exactly what the rewards were other
than knowing they were helping someone or knowing they were "doing
the right thing." As I left the graduation ceremony, I had absorbed
enough of this feeling to journey forward with a sense of quasi-religious
fervor about what I was about to do. Although I still felt a natural degree
of uncertainty, I realized that the training had provided us with some
knowledge, but perhaps more significantly it had instilled in us a belief
that the hospice way was "the right way." Our commitment to volunteering would probably depend a great deal on our continued faith in
the organization and that we knew how to "do the right thing" once we
met our patients.

In these first two chapters, I have presented the story of what
prompted me to become a hospice volunteer, what I learned about the
hospice movement from reviewing the literature about its history, and
the preparation I received for my role as a hospice volunteer. As I suspected from my earliest informal discussions about hospice, the word
hospice has many meanings. It is a philosophy of end-of-life care, as
well as a type of organization that provides a distinct system of services;
it can also refer to a specific place, such as LifePath Hospice, in which individuals give and receive these services. The word hospice always resonates with multiple connotations. Guided by principles of narrative
and ethnographic practice, for this research I immersed myself in the
culture of LifePath Hospice, to learn about being with someone who is
dying, and to narrate my experience of the hospice training, including
my thoughts and feelings as I learned about caring for dying patients
and what to expect from hospice volunteer work.

PART II

Entering the Country of the Dying

... death, the undiscovered country from whose bourn no traveller returns.

(*Hamlet*, Act III, Scene 1, lns. 78–80)

Among those who write about health and illness, geographical metaphors communicate the quality of a journey or quest that accompanies the progress of illness and treatment, and also the idea of separation or estrangement from others or from our own bodies (Geist-Martin, Ray, & Sharf, 2003). The metaphors of the body as territory (Frank, 1991) and illness as a country (Ellis, 1995b; Morris, 1998; Sontag, 1990) have a dual impact on our framing of the illness experience. The idea of travel can help to frame illness as a transitional state wherein we are "just passing through" and the idea of a country can separate us from others who are in the "land of the well." As I will discuss in the reflections at the end of Part II, one important lesson to keep in mind when communicating with people at the end of life is that we all hold "dual citizenship" (Sontag, 1990, p. 3); we will all become ill at some point, and we will all die some day.

I use the metaphor of "the country of the dying" to frame the stories in Part II because the initial stories from my visits with my patient and from the other volunteers reveal much of the naiveté, trepidation, and excitement of beginning a journey. In the title for this chapter, I employ the phrase "the dying" somewhat ironically—nowhere else in the book do I use those words to describe hospice patients. At this stage of the study, however, the other volunteers and I tended to have only a very generalized sense of who we would be visiting, how these patients would feel, and what it would be like to enter their world for a few hours every week. Composed of three chapters, many of the initial experiences described in Part II reflect a shedding of stereotypes and expectations about the dying, and a realization that hospice patients and their families would be as varied and as unpredictable as people in other contexts.

Chapter 3 recounts the first days of meeting and visiting my first patient. These visits illustrate the awkwardness of negotiating my interaction with her so that I could fulfill the hospice mission of "enhancing the quality of her life." Chapter 4 introduces the 6 volunteers who were the focus of the interview portion of the study—Sara, Emilia, Tom, Chris, Shyanne, and Hannah. The names of the volunteers and names in the narrative are pseudonyms; for those who are curious to know more about the methods of my study, I provide information in the Appendix about the interview process, the narrative, consent, and confidentiality. The six interview stories in chapter 4 describe our impressions of the training, our expectations, and our first visits to our patients. Chapter 5 returns to my narrative of visiting with my patient and describes the breakthrough that occurred once we started our routine of going out to lunch together. At the end of chapter 5, I present reflections on a significant dimension of starting hospice volunteer work— namely, the importance of facing the stereotypes and stigma associated with death and dying. Although each volunteer came to hospice with a different degree of experience and different fears about volunteering, all of us needed to transition from a generalized cultural understanding of death to an understanding based on the uniqueness of the individual patients and families we met.

3

Taking the First Steps

THE TELEPHONE CALL

Four days after graduating from the hospice volunteer training, my phone rings.

"Hey, lady! It's Norma from hospice." Her voice is as bright and enthusiastic as the first time we met. "How are you doing?"

"I'm doing fine," I reply, both excited and nervous. I remember feeling this way as an actor on opening night. All the preparation and visualization leading up to the performance could not eliminate the jitters of doing it for real.

"Listen," Norma continues, "I have a patient for you, if you're interested."

"Wow," I reply, "That's really quick."

"We have so many people waiting, we don't mess around!" Norma laughs. "If you decide to take this patient, I'll send you the notes in the mail, but in the meantime, you may want to write this down. Do you have a pen and paper handy?"

"Yes," I snatch a pen from my desk and pull my message pad toward me, "go ahead."

"Her name is Dorothy Samuels and she's 77 years old. She lives with her daughter, Terry Holmes, who is 52, and Terry's husband, Len, who is 56. Her primary diagnosis is end-stage COPD; do you remember what that means? Chronic, Obstructive, Pulmonary Disease—it's like emphysema. She's had a previous heart surgery, but that's all her chart says about her condition." Norma provides many more details about Mrs. Samuels—address, phone numbers, family history, dates, places, and names—and I soon realize that my message pad is inappropriately small for the task.

Norma continues, reading from her notes, "Dorothy's husband died 10 years ago, and Dorothy moved to the apartment complex about 2 years ago. Dorothy's daughter and son-in-law moved in 2 months ago, but it doesn't say where they lived before that. Terry was a bank teller but is not working right now. Len is a long-distance truck driver and he is continuing to work, which means he is on the road most of the time. Terry is the primary caregiver and will benefit from respite opportunities. The social worker has written here that both patient and caregiver are very receptive to hospice resources."

I guess that includes me. "Did Mrs. Samuels ever work?" I ask.

"Yes," Norma replies. "It says she was a cook. That's all I know."

"So, what can I expect regarding her COPD?" I ask. I remember passages from Final Negotiations, Carolyn Ellis's (1995a) story of taking care of her partner who had emphysema. I wonder how similar my experience with Mrs. Samuels might be. From what I learned during the training, I'm sure Mrs. Samuels will be using oxygen at this stage, and I'm glad we spent some time talking about how to deal with that. What I don't know is whether she'll be able to walk, or how breathless she may be. I want as many details as possible to prepare myself.

"She will be on oxygen," Norma confirms, "and hospice has ordered a wheelchair for her, a hospital bed, a shower chair, and a walker. I really don't have anything else to tell you about her condition. She can't drive, probably because she gets lightheaded and could faint, but her notes don't indicate that she has any problem walking, yet."

"Okay," I finish scribbling this last piece of information. I try to identify more questions to ask. A thought flashes through my mind and I say, "You didn't mention her race."

"She's white," Norma replies.

I feel a little disappointed, then, quickly reframe what I realize is a false assumption. As I imagined my first patient, I assumed it would be more challenging to volunteer for someone of an ethnicity different from mine and also more appealing because it would represent a greater learning opportunity. However, as I look over the details that Norma has provided about Mrs. Samuels, I realize that even though we are both white, there may be plenty of other cultural differences that we will have to negotiate.

I ask, "Is there a particular reason why she wants a volunteer?"

"Apart from providing respite for her daughter, I think the most important thing will be having someone to talk to, and something to break up the monotony of her day," Norma pauses for a moment. "So, what do you think? Shall I send you her information?"

"Yes … Absolutely!" I appreciate that Norma did not assume I would say yes.

"Great! I'll let Mrs. Samuels know that I've found someone and that you'll be calling to make an appointment. You can wait until you receive these notes and then call her, but I wouldn't leave it more than a couple of days."

"Okay." My head is spinning a little. I'm glad I have a day to wait for the patient notes.

"You know that you can call me any time," Norma reassures me. "You have all my numbers so if you have any questions, just call, okay?"

"Okay," I say, again.

"You'll be fine," Norma says, warmly. "Just make the first visit a short one to introduce yourself, then give me a call to let me know how it went, okay?"

"I will," I reply. "Actually, I'm already feeling nervous about it, but this is what I asked for, right? This is why I became a volunteer in the first place, to visit patients!"

"That's right," Norma responds. "You'll be great. It's always a bit nerve-racking meeting somebody for the first time, but you'll get over that."

After this conversation, my mind starts fantasizing about what my first visit will be like, then about what sort of a person Dorothy Samuels might be, and what our relationship will become. I wonder if she'll be like my grandmother. I wonder what we will have in common. When Mrs. Samuels's notes arrive 2 days later, of course they do not provide the answers to any of the questions that run through my mind. I want to know if she'll like me, if I can make a difference in her life, how long she will live after I become her volunteer, and if I will grieve when she dies. I can only learn the answers to these questions over time, by being with Mrs. Samuels and becoming a part of her life as she becomes a part of mine.

A few days later, I speak to Mrs. Samuels for the first time.

Terry answers and as soon as I introduce myself and ask for Mrs. Samuels, Terry hands over the phone saying, "It's someone from hospice."

"Hello, this is Dorothy."

Her voice is clear, cheerful.

"Hello, Mrs. Samuels. My name is Elissa and I'm calling because hospice told me you might like a volunteer."

"Sure, that sounds fine," she replies.

Mrs. Samuels's response surprises me because it sounds as though she wasn't expecting me to call. I press on. "Okay, well, I was wondering if I might come by on Tuesday next week; would the morning be good for you?"

"Any time," she says, brightly, "I'm usually here."

"Great," I hesitate for a moment, wondering if there should be more conversation. "Well, I'll call on Monday night to make sure that's still okay for you."

"You don't even have to call," Mrs. Samuels tells me, "you can just come by."

"Thank you," I pause, not wanting to reject her hospitality by insisting that I must call because of hospice regulations. Instead, I say, "I look forward to meeting you."

"Me, too," Mrs. Samuels says, warmly. "See you then."

We exchange goodbyes and I hang up the phone with a smile and a sigh of relief. That was not as hard as I thought; Mrs. Samuels's cheerful voice has infused me with optimism.

MEETING DOROTHY

After calling Terry and Mrs. Samuels yesterday to confirm my visit, I leave early to find their apartment. I have already checked the map, but the directions Norma provided are complicated. Sure enough, I find the location easily, but then drive around the entire property twice before I see where the numbers are posted on the buildings. The buildings are blocks of six or eight units, linked by covered breezeways in the middle so that the apartments have a kind of shared porch between them—not private, but certainly helpful to alleviate the heat of a Tampa summer. When I spot the number I am looking for, I cannot tell which breezeway to enter to find the apartment, and decide the only way to find out is to explore on foot. I park my car and am faced with a dilemma regarding my identification badge and the carry bag that LifePath provided for me—complete with a bright purple hospice logo. I have to wear my badge to identify myself, but I'm also supposed to protect the privacy of my patient and not let the neighbors know I'm from hospice. There are several groups of people sitting outside their doors, or on the steps of the buildings, or walking to their cars. I decide to carry my bag with the hospice logo against my body, and hold my badge in my hand until I'm right in front of the door.

As I walk through what I soon realize is the wrong breezeway, I note that I am unduly nervous about knocking on the wrong door. I straighten my shoulders and tell myself, "I'm from hospice. I'm a professional (sort of) and I know what I'm doing (sort of)." It takes me about 2 minutes to find the right place, but it feels like forever. Standing in front of the door, I clip on my identification badge, knock, and recall the introduction I imagined on my drive over here. I plan to extend my hand and say, "Hi, I'm Elissa Foster. I'm a hospice volunteer. You must be …."

The door opens abruptly and a fair-haired woman in her 20s appears in front of me wearing jeans, a tank top, and bare feet. Clearly, this woman is too young to be either Mrs. Samuels or her daughter Terry. For a second, I'm sure I've come to the wrong place.

"You from hospice, too?" the woman says, glancing at my badge.

"Yes," I reply, feeling startled and somewhat confused. "I'm the volunteer."

"Come in," she says, and holds the door open for me.

I step into a dark room filled with heavy furniture. The blinds are closed and there are two lamps providing a yellowish light. In addition to the young woman who opened the door, I see an older woman I assume to be Terry sitting on a sofa, and Mrs. Samuels sitting in a chair in the corner having her blood pressure taken by a hospice nurse.

"Hi," I announce to the room, unsure whom I should address first. I turn to Terry and thrust out my hand, "I'm Elissa Foster. We spoke last night." So much for my gracious and professional introduction! I wonder why Terry didn't warn me that my visit would coincide with the nurse's.

"Hi," Terry says, rising from her seat to take my hand. "I'm Terry and this is my daughter, Leslie."

There's one mystery solved. "Pleased to meet you," I say and I shake Leslie's hand. Both Terry and Leslie are fair-haired, blue-eyed, and curvaceous. Terry's face is warm and motherly, and shows the signs of many years spent tanning. Leslie's face is attractive but not welcoming. I wonder if she is feeling protective of her grandmother, concerned about Mrs. Samuels's illness, or simply suspicious of hospice, and of me.

"I'll be done in just a minute and then you two can get acquainted," the nurse says over her shoulder. "I'm Jackie, by the way."

"Hi, Jackie," I say. I look past Jackie to smile at Mrs. Samuels. "Good morning Mrs. Samuels!" I say, wishing I could at least shake her hand.

"Well, hello there!" she replies, smiling widely. "You can just call me Dorothy, everybody does! Why don't you take a seat over there? I'll be done with all this business in just a minute."

"Thank you," I smile. There are two sofas in the room, and Terry directs me to the one opposite Dorothy's chair. The television is on and Leslie and Terry are alternately watching a courtroom show and listening for questions from the nurse. As Jackie proceeds with her examination, I watch Dorothy. She is probably about my height, 5 feet 4 inches, but she seems tiny because she is very slender, with fine features. Her eyes are a lively blue-green and she looks over at me regularly to smile. Her hair is white, straight, and cropped very short in a practical style. As I expected, she is breathing through a clear plastic tube that extends from her nostrils, across her cheeks, over her ears, then joins under her chin to a long line, which I assume winds to the oxygen machine I hear humming audibly in another room. I wonder how long it will take for me to stop noticing the tubes.

"That's it, all done," Jackie announces, folding up the blood pressure cuff and stuffing it into her bag.

"Did you know that she knew me before?" Dorothy asks me in an animated voice.

"Who did?" I ask, "You mean, Jackie knew you before?"

"Yes," Dorothy replies, "She was my hospice nurse before."

I'm confused, and wonder if Dorothy is, too, until Jackie explains. "That's right. Dorothy was in hospice 10 years ago when she had heart surgery. I was taking care of both her and Stan, but Dorothy graduated."

I remember that Stan was Dorothy's husband, and he died about 10 years ago. But I did not know that Dorothy was a hospice "graduate." Since I first heard that expression, I've wondered what it must be like to be told you're dying and then go on to live for many years. I wonder how she feels about being in hospice for a second time.

"I'll see you next week, Dorothy," Jackie says, as she stands and walks to the door. "Bye, Terry. Bye, Leslie." They return goodbyes as Jackie closes the door behind her.

"Why don't you come over here so you and Mom can get acquainted?" Terry invites me onto the sofa with her so I can sit closer to Dorothy, in the space where Jackie had been. The arrangement of the chair and sofa means that I am sitting between them, and I find it hard to direct my attention equally to both, but I try.

As I move across the room, Leslie tells Terry, "I'm going to watch T.V. in your room, okay?" and walks down the hallway. I wonder why she doesn't stay and join the conversation.

"So, do you like doing this kind of work?" Terry asks.

"Yes, I do," I respond. I follow Norma's advice and do not tell them that this is my first time visiting a patient.

"What do you do when you're not doing this for hospice?" Terry asks.

"I'm a student at the University of South Florida. And I teach there," I add, feeling as though that may be the simplest way to describe what my life is like and how I earn a living.

"Well, that's wonderful," Terry says.

"Yes," Dorothy replies. "Good for you."

"Why don't you tell me a little bit about yourself, Dorothy?" I quickly change the subject. "I hear that you used to be a cook."

"That's right," Dorothy says, "I've cooked for thousands. Cooked for soldiers at the army base, even cooked for students like you at the university."

"Which university?" I ask.

"Auburn, in Alabama," Dorothy says proudly.

"Wow," I say, happy that we seemed to be finding common ground so quickly. "So you all must eat well around here," I suggest.

Terry laughs.

"We do," Dorothy says, "but we don't eat here. I won't do none of the cooking in my own house."

"Really?" I ask, surprised.

"Never have, and never will," Dorothy says, firmly.

"Is that because you got sick of cooking?" I ask.

"No," Terry interjects, "she's convinced that it costs more to drive and buy the groceries, bring them home ...."

"... use the utilities to cook everything and do the dishes," Dorothy concludes. "You may as well just go out to eat."

"Huh," I nod, though I'm unconvinced. "I guess so," I say to Dorothy. I don't want to contradict her right away, particularly since she seems so adamant about her logic.

Terry adds, "But don't think that we go out all the time. There is cooking going on in this place since I moved in here, right Mom?"

"Yes, she cooks, if that's what you want to call it!" Dorothy says, rolling her eyes in mock disgust.

Terry gives her mother a bemused look, then says, "Excuse me while I go and make some phone calls." She walks down the hallway to the bedroom.

Once we're alone, I say, "Well, Dorothy, I won't make this a long visit this morning, but I wanted to talk with you a little about what we might be able to do together for fun."

"I don't really know," Dorothy says. "I haven't really thought about it. What do you usually do?"

I don't *usually* do anything, I think to myself, feeling like an imposter.

"Do you have any hobbies?" I ask. "Do you like movies? I see you have a video player, perhaps I could bring some films over and we could watch them together?"

"I've never been one for movies," Dorothy replies. "Don't see the point of them. And I never had time for hobbies, I was always working, you see?"

"I understand," I reply.

"I like watching game shows," Dorothy says, brightly. "That's about the only thing I really enjoy on the television."

I nod and smile, thinking of how much I *dislike* game shows while trying to remember the suggestions they gave us at hospice. What am I going to do if there's nothing we can enjoy together?

"I'd be happy to watch games shows with you," I reply. "But is there anything else that you like to do for fun?" I ask. "Or something that I could help you with that you wouldn't otherwise get to do?"

Dorothy thinks for a minute and then smiles enthusiastically and says, "I do like to go out to eat. Maybe we could eat together some time?"

"Sure," I reply, "I guess we could do that some time."

After the training, when we had to nominate our preferences for volunteering, the one thing I wrote down that I *didn't* want to do was anything that involved transporting patients. As I think about going out with Dorothy, my mind fills with images of my car breaking down and of Dorothy having a heart attack in a restaurant somewhere. Ideally, I'd like to discover something fun to do here in Dorothy's home.

Dorothy's voice brings me back to attention. "And I used to like to go fishing with Stan, my husband," she says.

"I'm afraid I don't know anything about fishing," I say. "But perhaps we could take a drive to the water, and maybe you could teach me something?" It occurs to me that if Dorothy wants to get out of her apartment I want to make that happen for her, which means I need to address the sources of my anxiety. I mentally plan some repairs to my car and a call to Norma to review hospice guidelines for transporting a patient with COPD.

"I could teach you all about fishing!" Dorothy laughs. "Bait the hook, cast the line, pull in the fish ... nothing to it."

"Sounds great!" I say, still worried about my old car's ability to take us anywhere without breaking down. "Where did you go fishing with Stan, Dorothy?" I ask, initiating a brief conversation about the various fishing spots around town, none of which are familiar to me.

Dorothy and I chat together for about 10 minutes before Terry returns. She smiles, "How are y'all doing out here?"

"Fine," I reply.

"Just chatting with the babysitter," Dorothy winks at me and teases Terry with a gruff voice. "You don't need to check up on me. I'm well supervised, thank you very much!"

"Ha!" Terry addresses me, "You're already starting to see the ornery old lady inside the sweet little Grandma."

"I guess so," I smile. I've been here for around 45 minutes, and I recall that Norma suggested that I keep the first visit short. After a few more exchanges with Dorothy and Terry, I find an appropriate moment to say, "It's actually time for me to go for today. But I wanted to make sure this time is okay for me to come next week. I can certainly change days if this is going to overlap with your nurse's visits."

"You come any time you want to," Dorothy says. "I'm always sitting here, in this chair, staring at these four walls."

Terry says, "Jackie just changed days this week. I think she usually comes on Wednesdays, so Tuesday morning will be fine."

"Okay then," I reply as I stand. "I'll give you a call on Monday night next week to remind you that I'm coming."

"Thanks, Elissa. Is that right?" Terry checks her pronunciation of my name.

"That's right," I respond. "See you next week, Dorothy." I walk toward her and extend my hand. Dorothy seems surprised but clasps my hand and smiles brightly.

"Bye!" Dorothy says as I turn to leave. "You be careful now. There are all kinds of crazy drivers out there!"

"And thank God you're not one of them, Mom!" Terry says, good-naturedly.

"I'll be careful," I say, "I promise."

AN EARLY CRISIS

After my third visit with Dorothy, I walk into my apartment and immediately call the LifePath offices.

"This is Norma."

"Norma, it's Elissa," I say.

"Hi, lady!" Norma replies shifting from her professional tone of voice into the one that tells me I'm special. I love that Norma can communicate that feeling to me so easily, and I'm sure all her volunteers feel the same way—totally appreciated. "How's it going?" she asks.

"Terrible!" I wail.

"Why? What happened," Norma says, suddenly concerned.

"I think my patient's going to fire me! I'm a terrible volunteer!" I declare.

"She's not going to fire you!" Norma laughs warmly at my melodramatic announcement. "Why don't you tell me what happened?"

"Well," I begin, "I had my third visit with Dorothy today, and I'm convinced I'm going to bore her to death. Seriously!"

"No, you're not!" Norma says, and laughs again.

I continue, "We have nothing in common. She's really not interested in anything about my life—like school, or that I'm from Australia—and I try to ask her questions about her life, but I get confused really easily because she tells me these stories and there are so many names to remember. And I start to feel self-conscious about asking her questions continuously. Then today," I feel my insides cringe with embarrassment at the memory of it, "we were in the midst of a lengthy lull in the conversation and I saw a game of checkers on the table. So, I say, 'I see you have a checkerboard, Dorothy, would you like to play a game?' I remembered that was one of the suggestions in the volunteer handbook—playing cards or board games."

"Right," Norma prompts. "So what happened?"

"So, Dorothy says, 'Sure,' and we set up the board and in about 3 minutes, I can tell she has absolutely no interest in playing checkers. In fact, she started to look at her watch. So, after a little while, I said, 'We don't have to finish the game if this isn't fun for you, Dorothy.' And she said, 'Well, I thought you wanted to play,' and I didn't know what to say! I only suggested it because I thought it was something *she* might like to do. I don't even really know how to play checkers. It was awful, Norma!"

"It doesn't sound like you did anything wrong," Norma reassures me. "You have to remember that this is a *relationship*. It takes time for two people to get to know each other. You're not always going to 'click' right away."

Of course she's right, I think. Here I am, an interpersonal communication scholar, and I have completely unrealistic expectations about what my relationship with Dorothy should be like at this point in time. We don't know how to read each other yet, and it was silly of me to think that it would fall into place so quickly.

"Did you ask her what she would like to do for fun?" Norma asks.

"Yes," I'm feeling pessimistic and my tone of voice reflects that negativity. "She doesn't like movies, she has no hobbies, she doesn't play games, and she doesn't like shopping unless there's something specific she wants to buy. She did say that she likes to go out to eat, but she already does that with her daughter Terry, so I don't know how that will contribute to her life!"

"Maybe she would just enjoy going out with someone different," Norma says, sensing my impatience. "Give it time!"

"You're right," I reply. "It just feels so awkward when we run out of conversation."

"Maybe you would both feel more comfortable having something to do while you're still getting to know each other," Norma says. "Why don't you offer to take her out somewhere next week? What's the worst that can happen?"

"My car could break down and Dorothy could have a heart attack in the restaurant," I reply, morosely. "Or it could be really awkward again. I don't know which would be worse."

Norma laughs, "Elissa! Everything will be fine; Dorothy will have her oxygen with her. If you're worried about emergencies, you have all my numbers and all you have to do is call. There's no reason to think anything bad will happen, but if it does, you're not alone, alright?"

"Okay," I reply. I still feel afraid, but I also know that I'm inventing the terrible scenes that run through my head. Norma is right when she says there's no reason to think that something bad will happen. In fact, it makes more sense to imagine the best possible outcome. It would certainly put me in a better frame of mind.

"If you want," Norma says, "I can call Dorothy's nurse to make sure it's okay for Dorothy to go out. If she's still able to walk and you have her oxygen, then it should be fine."

"Thank you, Norma," I say.

"You're welcome," she replies. "Call and let me know how it goes, okay?"

After hanging up the phone, I look at the clock in my kitchen and realize that I only have a couple of hours before I conduct my first interview with Sarah, the young woman I met entering the LifePath building on the first day of the training. I am tempted to ask for her advice, but I also want to step back from my own experience, at least a little, to invite Sarah to tell her story.

4

The Volunteers' Stories

SARAH

From the first time she spoke to the group at the training, it was clear that Sarah was highly intelligent and passionate about her work as a graduate student in aging studies. She entered her doctoral program straight from her undergraduate degree, and was adamant that scholarship should be partnered with practical experience. She volunteered for hospice to experience the lives behind the cases and statistics that she studied. Because of her passion for integrating learning and lived experience, Sarah is definitely a woman after my own heart. At the beginning of our interview, Sarah explains that her academic interests are grounded in her personal history of witnessing her grandfather's experiences of cancer and Alzheimer's disease. As someone who has always been active in the community and volunteer work, Sarah's decision to become a hospice volunteer emerged naturally when she moved to Tampa to begin her studies and came into contact with the medical director at LifePath Hospice.

We are sitting in Sarah's office in the Aging Studies Department. She explains, "Hospice is more personal than the volunteering I've done before; most of it was general volunteer work in a nursing home. There were patients I got close to and spent time with, but this is the first time my volunteer work is based on visiting one person over an extended period of time." The distinction Sarah makes between the nursing homes and hospice is similar to my experiences in hospitals, where personal contact was never the focus of my duties as it is with hospice.

We talk a little about the training. We had both looked forward to becoming "trained" volunteers, but I confess to Sarah that I felt more nervous after graduation than I did when we began.

Sarah nods affirmatively. "I liked the training because they didn't tell you how to handle volunteering. They were honest in saying you have to go in there and see what happens. I hadn't thought about how close some of the relationships with patients would be. From my experiences in the past, people were reserved and there were issues they didn't raise. At the end of the training I wondered what I was going to be exposed to—aspects of people's lives that I wasn't sure I was ready to hear, and I questioned if I was the right person to hear them."

As we begin to talk about our patients, it becomes apparent that Sarah and I are facing similar situations. We are both visiting patients in their homes, and they are women in their late 70s who have chronic rather than acute conditions. Because of her expertise, Sarah has picked up on the implications of this far more quickly than I have.

"At my last visit, I talked to my patient about the fact that she could potentially be around for a very long time even though she's a hospice patient. Her heart's functioning at 50%, but 50% is pretty standard for chronic heart failure, considering that there are some people who live with 7 or 10% for a long time. I see this all the time, where people don't go into hospice at the right time. Time of death can be really difficult to predict, but even the hospice nurse said she thinks my patient could potentially be around for years."

I wonder if Dorothy could also "be around for years" and, if so, what does that mean in terms of end-of-life care? When Norma first mentioned graduation, I thought it was rare, but Dorothy graduated from hospice once before, and the same could happen to Sarah's patient. I wonder what we offer our patients if it isn't support and comfort for the last phase of their life.

I share my thoughts. "My patient has end-stage COPD. She's on oxygen, but to me she seems incredibly robust. I think her biggest problem is boredom because she's more or less confined to the house. We haven't talked about anything to do with end-of-life issues, and it's made me wonder what my role is in her life."

Sarah explains that her patient's daughter requested a volunteer for her mother. "I think she was concerned about her being lonely and having people to talk to. Although she has her family members and a couple of neighbors, her daughter wanted to introduce somebody else who doesn't know everything about her already, so she can talk more about who she is and where she came from. From day one, she's told me all about herself, the family members she's taken care of, her brothers-in-law, her brothers, and her sisters. So I think my role is just to listen, and to let her retell her life story, and to share with her little aspects of mine."

Sarah smiles and shakes her head a little. "And she likes to talk! She never lets the conversation lull. Her family concentrates on the illness; I get the impression that every time they call they ask how she's feeling. I think she just wants somebody around who doesn't talk constantly about what she's feeling and what she's doing, and doesn't harp on her about what she ate for dinner the night before.

"She said this is far from what she expected. She had surgery last November and she had no clue there was even a problem until January. So, perhaps it's still so new for her family that they haven't adjusted to it yet. I can be the person who doesn't make her think about it—a distraction from thinking about how sick she is."

It sounds as though Sarah and her patient have already established a comfortable and easy relationship. I recall the game of checkers with Dorothy earlier today, and wince. Trying to put it out of my mind, I ask, "How do you feel about your relationship with your patient? Do you feel like you're getting to know her?"

"Yes, I do, because she's so open and she's been through a whole lot in her life—and listening to someone is just important. The older you get, whether it's with someone in your own family or not, it's important that people get to tell their story before they pass. In her case, this is her chance to tell her story and I do look forward to seeing her because ...."

Sarah pauses for a moment and then continues. "I always leave there kind of tired, actually, which I didn't expect. I'm there for a good 2½ hours by myself and then her daughter comes home and, out of politeness, I stay for another half hour. But I'm there for close to 3 hours, and I leave there and I'm like—whew!"

It's reassuring that Sarah feels tired after visiting her patient. I am also exhausted when I leave Dorothy. Something about sustaining my attention and concentrating on her leaves me feeling drained. I file the observation in the back of my mind, and ask Sarah what her goals are for volunteering, and what she feels she is getting from it:

"Knowing that I'm helping—that in the midst of all this research, all these numbers and words that I put down on paper, sending things out for publication, I'm doing something that's actually helping somebody." Sarah gestures vigorously toward the surrounding offices. "Because I'm surrounded by these academics who are so out of touch with the real world—they just are!" Sarah catches me smiling at her small outburst and chuckles a little before continuing.

"It's also grounding. It reminds me on a regular basis that the little bitty bubble of people around me are far from the average person. Gerontologists, and psychologists, and all these aging-related researchers—they haven't seen an old person in 20 years! I think that's sad. I don't want to be one of those people. So, the personal connection with someone is important, and the most important thing is that it reminds me of what most people's lives, normally, are like.

"You can spend your whole life complaining about everything that you don't have, compared to what other people have. It's good for me to interact with people who were not raised the way I was; it gives me a greater appreciation for where I am and what I'm doing. Until you meet somebody who is 65 and has lived her life without an education, without even a high school diploma, you don't realize that where you're going is completely different."

Again, I see Sarah's reflections echoing many of my own. "I agree completely. I've realized that all the things I use in my daily life to get by—my degrees, teaching at university—they don't mean anything when I'm face-to-face with my hospice patient."

Sarah says, emphatically. "Those are the things that surprise me. Who I am and what I do are the first things out of my mouth—and this lady doesn't care. I'm there to talk to her and to visit with her, and where I'm in school and what I'm studying are irrelevant. I like that because it forces me to look at other parts of my life that define who I am besides my academic self."

I pick up Sarah's thread. "I do like that aspect of this work—getting down to basics. But it's one thing to know theoretically what to expect and it's another thing to be faced with an actual person and think, 'I have nothing in common with her! How can we possibly talk?' But for you, obviously, you've found something in common. How do you do that?"

Sarah shrugs slightly. "My guess is you just find something. If she mentions something I have no knowledge of, I ask her more questions. It makes her feel like she's teaching me something, sharing what she knows, and that there's something that we can both relate to."

It sounds like good advice, but I'm not sure it's always that easy. I respond, "At this point in my relationship with Dorothy, I'm aware that I'm looking to her to see if she approves of me and I think she's testing me out, too. 'How much can I tell you? How safe am I with you?' Maybe that's why you get tired after 3 hours? I do, too! I didn't expect to be as tired as I am."

"Definitely," Sarah agrees, enthusiastically. "When I go home, I'm like, 'Okay!' Even if I have errands, I just want to go home."

Partly because this is the first interview I conducted, and partly because so many of our experiences are similar, I leave this meeting with Sarah feeling reassured. I had imagined that I was the only person having doubts about what to do with a patient or struggling to maintain a conversation. Sarah appears to have fallen into step with her patient more quickly, and she is less worried, but her experiences suggest that my visits with Dorothy are not as far off track as I thought they were. By checking my perceptions with Sarah, I feel a sense of validation that helps me to have fewer doubts about my ability to be a good volunteer for Dorothy.

EMILIA

I liked Emilia immediately. At the training, she was very open and had no qualms about asking questions or expressing how she felt. Emilia is Brazilian American, 28 years old, and works as a graphic designer. Although she has lived in the United States for many years, Emilia's soft Brazilian accent flavors her speech deliciously. She is bright, beautiful, and creative—to all appearances, the girl with everything. Soon after we begin our conversation, she discloses that she lost her mother to lung cancer a year ago and, although her mother did not use hospice services, Emilia sees volunteering for hospice as a way to alleviate the pain of her own loss by helping others.

Emilia explains, "When you go through a loss, at least in my experience, and it may be temporary, but you see what's truly important in life. So, the nurses who were there, the phone calls, meant the world to me. It makes me cry even now to think about it, because if somebody even touched my hand or my mother's hair while I was at the hospital …." Emilia shakes her head gently, then continues, "If that had so much impact on me, maybe I could do that for somebody else. I could give a little back and, at the same time, deal with what happened."

Emilia describes her process of grieving and coming to terms with her mother's death. She cherished any contact from others that reminded her of her mother or gave her more insight into her mother's past. Once, Emilia received an e-mail from a friend of a friend—someone who had only recently heard that Emilia's mother had died. It simply said, "I remember your mother from college, the way she would drive around in her convertible with her hair down, holding a cigarette." That note means a great deal to Emilia, probably because it contributes to her ongoing relationship with her mother by providing her with a new memory to cherish.

I suspect many people would fear the pain of experiencing loss again, so I ask Emilia how she feels about working in hospice. Even as I ask the question, I know that I worry about that myself. I don't want to put myself in the position of reliving my grandmother's death, especially if it means I'm unable to respond appropriately to my patient's family.

Emilia explains, "Personally, I don't want to forget. I think this is a good way to remember." Emilia thinks for a moment and then continues: "One thing that I agree with is the hospice philosophy. Death is a natural thing, and I do see that, even though my mother just passed away, I don't see it as some horrible thing that happened to me. If anything, it's a wonderful experience to see hundreds of people come to me and my sister to say, 'Your mother touched my life.' Things that I took for granted, now I appreciate. Maybe if I were in shock I'd say volunteering would be a bad idea. But I think my situation is a little different."

Shifting topics, we share our impressions of LifePath. Emilia observes, gleefully, "They *touch* us, like the patients! I don't know if you noticed, but they hug and touch and put their hand on your shoulder saying, 'Sweetie,' 'Honey.' I come from a Latin culture where you kiss and hug and there is no 'personal space.' Being in the United States, where people are so distant ...."

As she trails off, I add, "In Australia we're a lot more 'huggy' too."

Emilia laughs, "I think it's only here that they're not."

"Don't you find that, because it doesn't happen as much, people crave that physical touch so much more?"

"It's amazing. Like they were saying at the training—a touch, a smile. With my patient, she probably wonders what's up, but I give her a kiss every time I leave. I kiss her hand and she always laughs at me, just for kissing her."

Like most of the other volunteers from the training, Emilia elected to visit in nursing homes. When she submitted her preferences for volunteering, the only things she requested were to be given a patient who was a nonsmoker, and someone with whom she could have a conversation—but it hasn't turned out that way.

"My patient is 99 years old," Emilia begins. "She has internal hemorrhaging of some kind, but if she dies, she will die of old age. She's had a beautiful, long life. She's been at home her whole life and finally this past year she's been put in a nursing home because they can't watch her 24 hours a day. She has dementia.

"She thinks she's still at home, so we spend every visit looking for people. We sit at the end of the hallway, because she doesn't want to be in her room, and she sits with her purse and we wait for her sister or her daughter to come pick her up. She'll say, 'She'd better come, because if she doesn't, I'm going to kick her butt.' Then she'll laugh a little and say, 'I never keep people waiting.' Because her eyesight isn't good she'll ask me, 'Hey, do you see anybody coming?' And I'll say, 'No, I don't see anybody yet.'

"So, I push her in her wheelchair, up and down the halls; sometimes we go outside, pretty much in search of the family. Here and there we'll get a little bit of communication. I'll ask her about her daughter or her son, but it soon goes back to, 'I hope they know we're here.' So, she thinks she's going home."

I ask Emilia if her patient knows where she is. Her patient sometimes knows that she is in a nursing home and is often aware of her surroundings, but she doesn't realize she is living there. Rather, she believes she simply is waiting to be picked up by her family and taken home.

"I don't quite get it," Emilia says. "She doesn't understand my relationship to her. I tried to explain, 'Your nurse, Kathy, sent me here,' but I don't think she realizes I'm from hospice. She's aware of her age because once she broke down and cried and said, 'I have no idea what I'm going to do. I'm old. I'm alone.' But she snapped out of it and went right back to, 'Where is she?' Some days she's more nervous and some days a little less.

"I know that in hospice they said that sometimes you might see someone once or twice and it's quick. I'm thinking with her, due to old age ...." Emilia does not finish her thought, but continues, "My great grandmother lived to be 105, so this lady could go on forever—or maybe not. She's very, very sweet, though. I thought I'd be uncomfortable with her dementia, but I just want to hug her. She has no teeth, she wants to eat cookies the whole time—as long as they're soft it's okay. The crumbs go all over and it gets a little messy, but who cares?

"I usually ask her permission. I say, 'Do you mind if I stay with you while you wait for Susan and Lawrence, just to keep you company?' And she'll say, 'Sure!' And I'll say, 'Okay, I'll stay here and chat with you so you don't have to wait alone.' I don't know what to say. I have no strategies. I just go with the flow."

Emilia appears to know exactly what to say and do with her patient; "going with the flow" is what is required in this case. Emilia's feelings about her patient suggest that they are establishing a connection even though the interaction is nothing like what Emilia had imagined.

"The first time she asked me 10 times who I was, but she doesn't ask me that anymore. I have all the hospice paperwork, so I feel like I know her a little bit. I am a little uncomfortable physically because there is nowhere to sit, and I felt weird going in circles wheeling this lady around the same small space. But nobody cares. Last time, one of the nurses said, 'Wow, she really likes that—that you're pushing her around.' It's nice that he made that comment."

Emilia seems to have taken the limitations of her relationship with her patient very well, so I ask, "You initially wanted a patient more like your mother, so I imagine this is challenging for you. Do you have a sense of your relationship with your patient?"

"I do feel that I have a relationship with her. The time that I spend with her is sweet. I know that she didn't ask for me, her daughter did, for companionship. So, just the fact that her family knows that someone's going to visit her might have an effect on me. I don't remember who said this, but one of the speakers at the graduation mentioned that sometimes the volunteers come and say, 'I don't know the difference that I'm making.' Do you remember that? She said, 'Oh my God, if you only knew the difference that you make.' And sometimes I feel that way. I wonder if I'm really having any impact, and I think that's partly the difference between my patient and having somebody like my mother; I could communicate, and share some stories, and feel like, 'Wow, we had a meaningful conversation and maybe that made a difference.'

"But with this—it's nice, it's relaxing. In a way, it's like meditation. Because when I leave, it's like nothing matters. I sit there and I think, 'Wow! And I was worried about the dentist,' or whatever. So it's good for me. But I don't cry or feel emotional. It's like an empty feeling. Like I just stepped out of my own reality and came back. I just stopped for a while."

Later in the interview, Emilia returns to this theme. "I spend so much time thinking about myself. Then, with my patient, I have to step out of my world. I have to not be selfish. I have to say, 'Emilia, shut up. You're not here for you. It's not about *you*.' Like at work, you always want to put your two cents in, but here it doesn't count. It's not about me, and that's hard for me."

I agree. "I think sometimes it's hard for me, too, particularly since a lot of my life is spent teaching. What I say *does* matter in the classroom, and I'm secure in that authoritative teacher role. Now, I'm in a situation where somebody else is in the center, and I have to read her and decide, 'Is this working for her or not? Is she getting tired? What else can we talk about?'"

"And you're not the focus," Emilia adds.

"Right."

"So that's a lesson in itself. Originally—not that I thought I would come in and tell my life story—but I thought, 'Oh, somebody might be interested in *me*.' But it's not that at all. Who cares?! Like this lady. She does not know my name! I'm just this person, maybe like her little angel; I just show up and walk her around and leave. And I'm always smiling, and I take cookies for her. No relationship, don't know her family. I don't know what she thinks of me."

I confess that I don't yet know what Dorothy thinks of me either, and that it's driving me a little crazy. Emilia asks if there are any awkward pauses in the conversation. I say, "I feel like most of our time together is spent in awkward pauses!"

"So you have your own challenges," Emilia points out. "Because *you* need to think; *I* need to act. For me, it's 'Okay, let's go, let's go! We're on the move! In the wheelchair!'"

"Do you ever think about what it will be like when your patient dies?"

Emilia looks wistful as she thinks about my question. "I think with her I can see myself going to church, lighting a candle. Sometimes I sit and I laugh when I remember—not anything particular—just sweet little things. That will be in my heart, in my memory, and so it's not tragic in any way. So I think when she passes away I will say, 'Well, this lady had a beautiful life.' I know from the notes that she has a caring family. I totally understand why they placed her in the nursing home. It's sad, but it's her time. She's 99."

Emilia's responses makes me consider the complex motives that the volunteers have for volunteering. Although Emilia reminds herself often that she must put her patient's needs first, she also recognizes that hospice volunteering is helping her to reach personal goals. Emilia commented that tragedy can be a blessing in disguise, and her responses throughout the interview reveal a similar duality in our volunteer activities—we cannot separate the giving part of what we do from the receiving. This duality is part of every type of close personal relationship, except that the volunteer–patient relationship does not fit easily into that category. We have only just met our patients; we are not drawn together by similar interests or shared associations with other people. In Emilia's case, her patient may never learn her name.

Perhaps our consciousness of the intrinsic rewards of the volunteer–patient relationship, and our willingness to experience those rewards, make the relationship personal. Similarly, because our patients are at the end of life, we are aware that life is short, and perhaps that means we focus on the positive aspects of the experience, rather than the negative. I continue to toss these ideas around in my mind as I drive home from the interview.

TOM

The evening after my meeting with Emilia, I interview Tom. During the training, he impressed me as a warm and caring person. I know he works for an insurance company, but that is all I know about him. When we arranged the interview, I discovered that he lives in the most exclusive part of town. I pull into the parking area of his building and walk across the marble floor of the lobby to announce myself at the security desk. I am struck by the apparent disparity between the affluence of the building and Tom's approachability. I know I am engaging in inverted snobbery—an acknowledged cultural characteristic of Australians—but I can't help myself. I wonder what prompted Tom to journey from his very comfortable lifestyle into the world of visiting hospice patients in nursing homes.

Tom's warm welcome feels like I am meeting up with an old friend. Tom tells me he is in the process of moving from his apartment to a new home that he is building a few miles away. We talk for a little while about his move and Tom graciously shows me the view from his balcony, a gorgeous panorama of the city at night, which prompts me to ask about where he grew up. Tom discloses that he grew up in New York and Los Angeles, a real "city kid."

Once we settle in the living room, and my tape recorder is set up, I ask, "So, what brought you to the LifePath volunteer training?" He says he will give me the quick version, although I assure him that long stories are okay, too.

"About 3 years ago, I was listening to a radio program in the car late one night. There was a lady on the program who was a past-life regressionist—someone who hypnotizes people to discover who they were in a previous life. I bought her book and started reading other books about past-life regression. Then, I came across one book called *Saved by the Light,* written by a man who was struck by lightning. After this happened, he had visions of what he was supposed to do with the rest of his life. He felt he was supposed to start a program just like hospice. So, half of the book was about the program that he started, how it made him feel, and how he was helping people. Reading that book was what got me thinking about volunteering. Finally, about 6 months ago, I was moving to Tampa and I thought, 'Now I'm going to do it.' I got on the computer and I typed in 'hospice' and I put in 'Tampa' and LifePath Hospice popped up. I e-mailed them to say I was interested in volunteering, then I got the invitation in the mail 2 or 3 months later, and that's how I got there."

Tom's story surprises me. I'd expected to hear an account more like Emilia's, involving the loss of a relative. He didn't announce his interest in past-life regression at the training. Although there was an atmosphere of openness and acceptance at the training, Tom may have been concerned about how others might respond, or he may not have felt invited to talk about that aspect of his interest in hospice.

I want to make sure that I understand Tom correctly. "So, *Saved by the Light* made you interested particularly in being around people who are dying so you can learn from that?"

"Yes, I've read a lot about how some people leave in despair—but there's so much you can do for someone who is afraid or is getting ready to go and feeling really uncomfortable about things. You can help them feel better about it, or kind of like hospice says, just be there for them. So that's probably what my real intention was—to help people in that way. But I'm not so much interested in just being around them, but to see what they feel like and what they're thinking, to see if there were things I could say that would help them get through it a little easier.

"I used to have a great fear of death—an overwhelming fear of death. But in the last 3 years, from all the things I've read, death doesn't have the same negative effect on me that it does on most people. I can put that all aside and just have a conversation with someone who's dying. But I couldn't have done that 5 years ago."

Tom had decided to volunteer at a nursing home. He was partly persuaded by Patrice, and he also felt safer knowing that there would be someone "right outside the door" if anything went wrong. As we discuss our first visits, Tom speaks about what was difficult for him.

"Before the training, I thought about all the things that have happened to me over the last 3 years that I could talk to people about when I visit them. But after the training, I realized that's the opposite of what I should be doing. You're not supposed to explain your beliefs; you're supposed to listen to what they have to say." Tom chuckles, "Besides, a lot of people would find the kinds of things I think about to be a little 'off the wall.'"

"So, how did your first visit go?"

"I found the really hard part was being able to sit there and not talk. The person I'm seeing gets really tired, so I felt the need to keep the conversation going, and with her not contributing, the only thing I could really talk about was me. And I'm trying not to say things like, 'I'm building a house; it's really nice.' So, I was uncomfortable, trying to think of things to say that wouldn't make her feel bad or sad about the state she was in.

"But I remembered Patrice saying it's fine just to sit there and not say a word. So I said, 'Do you want me to leave? Because you look really tired.' And she said, 'No, I'm just tired. But I want you to stay.' So I sat there for 15 minutes. Neither one of us said anything. Every now and then she would open her eyes to see if I was still there."

"Did you hold her hand? Or are you not at that point yet?"

"Well," Tom tilts his head a little to one side, "when I first walked in she did not look well—not that I was expecting her to look great. It was a very nice nursing home, by the way, like a 5-star hotel. The downstairs was really pretty and then her room looked just like a hospital room; it was not homey at all. She was in a hospital bed lying on her side, and she looked really small. I had to lean down to the side of the bed so she could see me."

I note Tom's body as he tells me this story. I imagine his efforts to soften his presence so that his intrusion into her space was gentle and not intimidating, his tall, masculine frame stooping down toward the tiny figure in the hospital bed. When we met, his appearance struck me as almost teddy-bearish and I wonder if he knows that he makes that impression.

Tom continues, "It took a while to explain who I was. I said, 'Nurse Donna asked if I could give you some company.' Then, she asked me to come back another day because she was really tired. I said, 'Sure.' I was pretty close to her. She reached her hands out and so I reached down and held both of her hands in my hands. That was in the first 15 minutes and we were holding hands. But, she obviously wanted me to touch her because she reached out, which was truly an effort because she was really weak. Since then, I've visited a few times. When I went on Sunday she was like a different person. I could understand what she was saying a lot better."

I'm still smiling from Tom's lovely description of his first interaction with his patient. I probe further. "What did you talk about?"

"She loves gardening, so we talked about her garden and the flowers that she likes. On her windowsill she had all these little cups with twigs sticking out of them that she was trying to grow—and you could see that it just wasn't going to happen. She had a roommate and each of them had one of these big bulletin boards next to the bed. Her roommate's bulletin board was covered with grandchildren's pictures, but she didn't have anything on her bulletin board. I told her I would find some pictures of flowers for her to put up there.

"I go to London a lot, and I associate London with flowers, and they have all these gardening magazines there. So, I cut out all these pictures and brought them back with me from London last Sunday. I let her look at each one, then I put them up on the bulletin board until it was covered with flowers. We probably spent, seriously, 30 or 40 minutes talking about her garden—what kind of citrus trees she has, and apples and cherry trees. She told stories about her garden and she asked me about the weather and whether it was making the grass greener. You know it really struck me that she was thinking about the weather in terms of gardening rather than just 'How's the weather?' So, that's why I thought she would like them, and she really did."

"I'll bet she did love them! That's a wonderful story." I'm smiling broadly, and also feeling a little teary-eyed in response to Tom's story. "I have an image of you in my mind—we just looked at your urban view out the window. You grew up in New York City and Los Angeles, and you're with a patient who's interested in gardening! Do you have any experience with gardening to draw on or did you just ask her questions?"

"I asked her questions, and she's taught me quite a few things. I'm getting ready to do a lot of gardening. I have landscapers working at my new home now, so I'm thinking about asking her advice, particularly because there's a lot of sand down here."

I respond. "It's great that she feels comfortable talking about things that she has loved. And I just love that you thought to find pictures of flowers for her!"

Tom grins and nods. "They made her so happy. You know, I was a terror growing up in the Bronx, so this is just really new to me."

"So, were you cutting them all out yourself?" I ask, returning Tom's smile. In my mind, I can just see Tom, hunched over, concentrating on the delicate work of cutting out flowers from magazines—all for a woman he has only just met.

"Exactly. I was looking for the ones with the most colors. Now, I have to find some new ones because she's looked at those for a few days now. You know," Tom reflects, "I think her family is so used to her gardening that they wouldn't think to talk to her about it. With me she gets to relive that all over again, telling me how she planted apple trees in Maine, how old they are, how to pick grapefruit, how to know when something's ripe and when it's not. Like her flowers on the windowsill. She really knew what they all were!"

I reflect, "She becomes center stage. She's the star of the time you spend together."

Tom agrees. "She ran the conversation; she was the knowledgeable one. She wasn't when the nurse came in telling her what she needed, or some financial person, or a doctor. She got to take charge because she was the one with all the knowledge about gardening. That probably made her the happiest, to actually be in control of the conversation on a topic she enjoyed."

"You said something earlier about being with someone at this stage of life and expecting to have conversations about that experience. I can see that happening at some time with Dorothy, but I can also see going through this whole process and never talking about death, how she's feeling, or her fears. At first I was worried that I wasn't going to fulfill my job. But maybe talking about gardening, or sharing family stories ..."

Tom interjects, "I almost wouldn't want to talk to her about death and dying unless she wanted to. If that's what she wanted, I'm sure she would have found a way to bring it up, and we haven't even come close to the subject. If you really want to, you can ease your way around to a topic pretty easily. I didn't feel like I wanted to explain death to her or help her get through it."

"It's the difference of having it come from them rather than from us," I suggest.

"It's kind of a fishing expedition. We're going in there and we've got to find the right bait to catch them. If it's gardening or a movie or whatever, we have to fish around until we find it. Once we've found the thing that makes them happy to talk about, they'll open right up. After that, anything you want to talk about probably is fine with them because they really just want you to be there. You just have to find that first thing. That's how you can tell you've found it; they ease back and relax when they've found that topic they feel good talking about."

Tom's observations reveal details of his experience that are easy for me to identify with and seem so simple, and also express a complex 'intangible' regarding these early conversations with our patients. I smile, "That's a great analogy! Actually, my patient and I talked about fishing the first day I visited her. That's what I feel I've been doing, particularly these first few weeks. I'm throwing out the line and coming back with nothing! I guess I need to accept that she needs to get out of the house, while she still can." "It's good that you're doing this project," Tom says. "It probably helps you out a lot. You get to hear about all the different situations. For me, just listening to what's happening with your patient has got my mind thinking in different directions, and you're hearing it from everybody."

I agree. "It is great, because this group is very diverse and everyone has taken such different paths to get to the same place but there's something in all of us that brought us there. It transcends race and class and gender and everything."

Although it is getting late when I drive home from Tom's apartment, I feel excited and energized. Tom has given me a window onto some of the magical moments that can emerge in the volunteer–patient relationship, even in the early days of the relationship when communication is difficult. I wonder if Dorothy is interested in gardening.

As Tom pointed out, these conversations with the other volunteers are teaching me so much; I start anticipating the interviews I have coming up in a couple of days.

CHRIS

I have scheduled two interviews for today; the first is with Chris in the morning, and the other is with Shyanne just after lunch. Unlike the other volunteers, Chris is still waiting to be assigned to a patient, but I proceed with the interview because I want to know his reasons for volunteering. Chris and I sat together during the training and he made a big impression on me. Tall and slender, with a deep yet soft voice, Chris is in the social work program at the University of South Florida, and I judged him to be about 23 years old. At Chris's suggestion, we meet at the local library. Chris first describes his work as a funeral director, a fact I do not recall from the training. He says he has been licensed for about 15 years, working in the family business. Something doesn't add up.

"You seem really young to be a funeral director," I observe.

Chris smiles, "Actually, I turned 40 in February."

Unsuccessfully, I try to stop my jaw from dropping. "Congratulations!" I sputter, betraying my surprise.

"I'm middle aged—or heading there," Chris chuckles.

I feel myself revising my assessment of Chris. I am fascinated that this gentle, youthful man is a funeral director and am curious to know what he enjoys about his work.

"In planning a funeral service, you meet people at a point in their lives when everything has been turned upside down. The only thing they can count on at that point, as far as something material, is how their loved one will be presented at the service. When we restore their loved one so they appear as they were prior to sickness or whatever happened, one of the greatest things is the satisfaction of the family. Sometimes they tell us verbally, and other times they don't have to say anything, it just shows when they see their loved one. You can tell when they're pleased."

I am reminded of my colleague Christine's narrative ethnography (Kiesinger, 1999; Kiesinger, 2001), in which she describes assisting her brother, a funeral director, to prepare the body of a young woman she had known. The narrative describes the radically altered appearance of the woman's body, which had undergone an autopsy and—through a careless clerical error at the airport—been left to freeze outside the terminal. As Christine assists her brother, they return their high school friend to the appearance they remembered, sparing her loved ones from the shock they had experienced upon first seeing her. Hearing Christine's story, I realized for the first time what the restoration of a body could mean to family members. With this image of Chris's work in my mind, I turn my attention back to his story of coming to hospice.

"So this is your first contact inside hospice, to become a volunteer. Have you been thinking about it for a long time?"

"Yes. I've been thinking about it for quite a few years. But I've been concerned because, working as a funeral director, you have to be careful of getting involved with another business that's closely associated—like with nursing homes—that people don't jump to the conclusion that you're there to get business. Do you know what I'm saying?"

"Yes." I know so little about funeral homes that, had Chris not mentioned it, I would not have considered the potential conflict of interest between volunteering for hospice and being a funeral director. Chris says that he told hospice about his family's business when he signed up for the training, and I wonder if Patrice advised Chris not to mention it to the other volunteers. I can also see how someone like Chris, who is comfortable with the tangible manifestations of death, and familiar with grief, would make an ideal hospice volunteer. Chris also may have presented himself as a social work student because he received class credit for the training.

Chris explains, "My main interest in social work is to address the high incarceration rate of young people, mainly African Americans, because it *is* disproportionately greater than in the white population. I think as an African American male, and I have younger nephews and so on, it's on my conscience constantly. So, that's my main area of interest for my degree, but I wanted to use this class volunteering project to do something I have intended to do all along, and that is to get involved with hospice. In years to come, I may be putting most of my time into doing just the social work, and I won't be able to volunteer then."

I observe that Chris has a strong sense of social justice. He explains that his mother has influenced him greatly through her work with young people who come into contact with the court system, and a program she ran in the 70s that took African American children to visit New York and Washington. Then, Chris asks about my patient.

"I've visited Dorothy four times in her home," I respond. "For most visits, her daughter is there, and sometimes her granddaughter lives with them. We haven't had much time just one-on-one. We are trying to establish how I can make her life a little brighter. One thing I didn't feel secure about was transporting my patient anywhere, but that's really what she needs. There's no way that LifePath could have known Dorothy's need for outings from the assessment that they did. So, I got some additional information to feel okay about taking her out because she needs a wheelchair and portable oxygen. We're going out to a fishing pier next Tuesday."

"That's great," Chris smiles broadly. "And how old is she?"

"She's 77."

"That human contact, especially when you're getting older, is so important because that's what keeps the minds of seniors active. I believe it's unfortunate that everybody doesn't find themselves in their old age with a lot of family around. My father, he's 83; he's a retired teacher. That may be part of the reason why his mind is so alert, but another part is that he has these little grandsons that he takes to school every day. Most people think that he's in his 60s and it's like he's too busy to get old." Chris chuckles a little, "There's a lot to be said for not slowing down, not necessarily staying active in work, but just in life.

"At the hospice support meeting on Tuesday, Patrice described how they determine when to release someone from hospice care, and I asked her what, in older age, is the intended purpose of hospice? Do patients have to be terminal? I wondered if the older patients still need somebody coming to see them. People stay in better health when they have that contact."

I nod in agreement. "Yeah, that's a tricky question. I'm not medically trained, but my patient, Dorothy, occasionally has coughing fits that tell me her lungs are in really bad shape, but she's also very alert, and she doesn't have any trouble speaking. To me, she could go on and on. She just doesn't look like someone who's dying—not the way I expected anyway. It occurred to me that if they release her from hospice care and say, 'Well, you've improved sufficiently,' it would be awful. 'You've got to deteriorate again before we give you back your volunteer.'"

I am a little surprised that Chris brought this issue up with Patrice even though he has not yet seen a patient. I ask, "What kind of experience would you like to get from hospice volunteering? Obviously, you said you were with Patrice's group, the nursing home group, so ...."

Chris responds, "Whenever I'm having a first experience of something, I look at the situation and say, 'Since this is the first experience, then where would be the place where I might be most relaxed?' In the nursing home, you can concentrate on the experience itself; whereas, you have to be careful in someone's home because the protocol for behavior is different—not that I'm thinking about misbehaving," Chris smiles, "but it varies from home to home. In the nursing home, it's going to be pretty much the same situation wherever you go. The nurses are probably used to people coming in there, hospice coming in there. In the home, it may be their first time, too, and they have to get used to having a stranger in their home."

I think about Emilia's experience with her patient in the nursing home, and ask Chris: "Have you considered being with a patient who has dementia?"

"I've definitely thought about it. I think I mentioned at the meeting that I have an aunt with Alzheimer's. That's what they called it. I have a different theory about that. My aunt, she had these ways about her—she had an ornery type of attitude—but *dementia*? Once you understand *why* a person is reacting in the way that they are, they can be easy to understand."

I shift topics a little. "Hospice talks about the concept of holistic care—to the body, to the mind, and to the spirit. What do you think we bring to the hospice patient in that regard?"

"For one thing, as I said before, human contact is extremely valuable and you can't replace that with anything else. It keeps people alive. I guess without human contact, it would be like that saying, 'If a tree falls in the forest, and there's no one there to hear it, does it make a sound?' In that situation, someone is alive but there's no other human contact, so are they really alive? Are they experiencing life? So, the greatest thing about hospice is reaching a lot of people in their homes, who are sick or shut in, or who have no other contact."

Chris pauses as a group of children walk past us in the library. They are tiny, and trying to be very good as they walk hand-in-hand, elephant style, past the table where we are sitting and toward the door. I can't help smiling at them all.

"They couldn't be more than 2 or 3 years old," I observe, struck by the contrast. "It's amazing. We're sitting here talking about the end of life, and we're passed by a little crowd of newbies—new to the world!"

"Yeah!" Chris smiles, too. "And that's another thing with hospice, sometimes we have to deal with kids and their lives ending. That's something in the funeral business we have to deal with that's very difficult, the death of children of any age."

Chris tells me about an experience that he had when he was in the fifth grade and lost two friends in a car accident. "I think to this day of all the things they never got to see, like the first personal computer and even VCRs, camcorders—mostly things that people in general are using these days. They never got to see them—not that that bothers them.

"That's one thing that people have to realize; we're the ones who have to deal with these things that come to our minds. It's like the funeral service; we put on the service for the living, not the dead. It's said in the Bible that the dead know nothing. If they *do* know something, we don't know *how* they know it, so it's irrelevant to us. But we do know that the living are affected by it, so that's what we're concerned with."

Chris's observation reminds me, "One of the things that the hospice movement talks about is the notion of the 'good death.' I don't know if you've heard of that."

"I heard Patrice mention that."

"Do you, yourself, have any kind of concept at this point of what that would mean? For you, as a hospice volunteer, being part of providing this good death?"

"The good death ..." Chris reflects for a moment. "That's an important concept. There can be a stress-free death when the person is ready to let go, and there's no feeling that they have to hope for something that might be hopeless as far as trying to live another day. For instance, with me, when that time comes, I don't want anything to keep me alive for *another minute* if there's no quality in it. So, I would like to prepare myself and go peacefully."

"Do you feel that you're providing spiritual care just by making contact with a patient; that there doesn't have to be anything more?"

"I think that certain acts are spiritual in nature. You're there for no other reason other than that person, so what else could it be? You're not being paid, so it's not financial. I would say it's spiritual. I think that's the main reason why I wanted to get involved anyway, to get more in touch with the spirit."

"That's a great way to think about it," I smile. "Hospice, it is an institution, a bureaucracy in and of itself, but they seem to have put a process together so that humanity remains. The more I talk to people, the more I think it's the volunteers who make it that way."

"I think it's the volunteers," Chris agrees. "If it weren't for the volunteers, if it were only those who were paid, I don't think you'd have the same situation because then profit comes into play. For example, when I go to visit someone, my time is so limited that if I don't leave at a certain time I'm going to have a big problem. At the same time, it's hard for me to say, 'I've made my time and now I've got to go.' That defeats the purpose of being there; a friend would not treat you like that, because friends aren't on the clock. So, if not for the volunteers, visits would be measured in dollars and cents, and I think you'd see a big difference. A lot of these people don't have others who are there for no other reason than they *want* to be there."

My conversation with Chris prompts me to reflect upon the value of simple, human contact, of quietly keeping company with someone, and paying attention to their presence. I try to remember the last time I felt lonely, or in need of company when there was no one to talk to. I've never realized the extent to which I take my social network for granted. I live with the assumption that there will always be people around me who know the details of my life and who care about the condition of my spirit, but that is not necessarily true. I think about Dorothy. She used to be surrounded by family, friends, and coworkers and now she spends her days, as she puts it, "looking at these four walls." Perhaps I should stop worrying about entertaining Dorothy, and learn to recognize and value the basic human connection that we experience together. As I make my way down to South Tampa to meet up with Shyanne, I think about next week's visit with Dorothy, and decide to plan a drive together. Perhaps she'd like to see the bay.

SHYANNE

Shyanne has a certain aura, a combination of grace and stability, which attracted me to her when we first met at the training. Shyanne also appears very serene and confident, and at first, I felt agitated and unfocused by comparison. When she introduced herself to the group at the training, I was impressed by the ease with which she spoke about how she had "issues with death," which she was attempting to confront through volunteering. She also acknowledged that she had lived a very blessed life, and that she wanted to give something back to the community. Two things about Shyanne stand out in my mind as I prepare to interview her. Like me, Shyanne immigrated to the United States from a Commonwealth nation—South Africa—and so I feel a connection with her as a fellow immigrant. Second, Shyanne is a counselor and works as a life coach—a profession I have always admired. I look forward to her unique insights into her experience of volunteering.

We meet at a small coffee shop on the south side of town, near where Shyanne lives in an older, picturesque neighborhood. When I locate the coffee shop Shyanne has suggested, it strikes a chord with me; it reminds me of home, and I wonder if she feels the same way.

We begin by talking about what brought us to hospice. Shyanne tells me that she was not exposed to death and dying growing up, so she never had an opportunity to think about it. Then, she shares a compelling story of the moment she realized she had a problem dealing with death.

"Six or 7 years ago, I was backing out of the driveway, and I was listening to a commentator talking about a comet; I can't remember the name of the comet, but it would only be visible again in the year 2080. So, I thought, 'Oh, 2080,' and suddenly, with a jolt, I realized that I wouldn't be here to see the comet when it came again. I went into a tailspin. I drove back up my driveway, went into the garage and sat there. After about an hour, my husband came and said, 'What's going on?' and I told him. I knew I had a problem. I hadn't realized before that I was going to die. It just hit me, at 35."

I ask, "This was about 6 or 7 years ago, this epiphany, and was that a catalyst for you to seek an active way of overcoming, or understanding, death?"

"Yes," Shyanne replies. "But first I started living life like there was no tomorrow. I went back to college, I got an MA degree, I started my practice and two support groups, we moved house, I got my husband into a different profession, we were traveling. I didn't want to rest for a minute in case I died if I sat down. After a few years, my husband said, 'Something's going on and you need to examine it; you're so caught up in living that you don't have time to think of death and there's a balance.' I was juggling and not balancing, and I felt hypocritical because, to my clients, I preach balance. I appeared to be this swan on the serene lake, the person who had it in control, the great life, gliding on this lake, while underneath the water my feet were going crazy. No one could see that except myself and my husband because he knows me so well. So I decided to quit being a swan. That was probably the hugest thing in my life, short of pledging my life to another human being and becoming a parent. That epiphany changed everything."

I think about the role that epiphanies have played in the lives of the volunteers. For some, it was a dramatic event, for others a sudden insight. All of us, at some point, took the step to volunteer for hospice. Whether we were aware of it at the time or not, I believe that our lives will be changed significantly by that decision.

Shyanne describes having read a magazine article by a woman who was dying. In the article this woman described what she didn't want her friends to do. "She was trying to tell her friends that she needed them to be real. She told them, if I look like crap, then say,' Let's go wash your hair,' or, 'Do you feel like taking a bath? I'll help you,' or 'What do you need me to do around this house for you?' She didn't need to hear, 'I know how you feel.'"

Shyanne leans forward a little. "So I wondered how I would deal with it if a friend of mine had a terminal illness. I felt that I wasn't equipped to honor that person with the skills that I had. At the bottom of the article was a Web site for hospice, and that site had a link to LifePath. So I called and said, 'How do I get involved?' My heart was pounding; I was clammy and sweaty. It was the beginning of the week and they said, 'We have training this weekend. Do you want to start?' It was a *huge* deal."

Given the challenge that hospice represents for Shyanne, I am curious to hear about her early meetings with her patient.

Shyanne begins. "I grew up in South Africa, and the whole apartheid issue is very sickening to me. I was raised to think of black people in a particular way, which is why I did not raise my children over there. I didn't want them thinking that way. So, my first patient is a beautiful black woman. She is 77 years old, she has breast cancer, and—I can't tell you—" Shyanne pauses, then says, "I see your reaction."

Sitting in the coffee shop, with only a very few words, Shyanne gives me insight into her experience and the poignancy of her situation catches me off guard. My eyes are tearing up.

Shyanne nods gently and continues. "That's how I felt. It's the most amazing thing that she's in my life and I can't wait to see her every time I visit her. She doesn't want much from me, either. It was a challenge for me, not only because of the black–white issue, but because I was raised in a very wealthy environment. I live a very comfortable lifestyle and I always have. I've never had to worry about where I live or money issues. And she lives in the projects, in the most squalid conditions you could ever imagine, in a scary neighborhood where people hear gunshots at night, and the cops are patrolling, and if you leave your car unlocked it's gone. So she lives locked in her dark, dingy, 2-room apartment, 24 hours a day, just afraid.

"I go there a couple of times a week and each time I say I'm only staying an hour or so, and I end up staying at least 2 hours. And it's so funny, because here's this skinny little white woman and here's this old black woman with an elementary school education, who's been a maid in a hotel all her life, who grew up in a terribly abusive household, knows what it's like to be hungry and poor. And yet, we instantly connected because we left out all the bullshit and connected on a human level. And we connect as two women—we can talk about men, our husbands, what society expects of us as women, and what we want out of life. I realized she shares the dreams, desires, and aspirations that I have. We're sisters under the skin. That really struck me."

I think about my visits with Dorothy. As I discussed with Sarah, although my patient and I are of the same race, I realized quickly that the things I feel are most important about me mean little or nothing to her. The fact that I am doing research, teaching at the university, or even that I come from Australia, are not things that she's curious about—and it perplexes me.

I tell Shyanne, "I'm a little intimidated. I wonder, 'Do I have what it takes to engage her, to be interesting to her?' Because my life experiences haven't matched hers."

Shyanne responds quickly. "But you judge yourself when you say that, and in some ways you're judging your patient, too. I think in our society we get so used to being these little human *doings*. You've been a human doing all your life, I'll bet, doing and going to school and teaching your classes. But you're a human being and that is what we give to our patients. Sometimes they don't even need us to give them any pearls of wisdom or to say anything: just a nod of the head or a smile, holding a hand, laughing at some silly joke that someone cracks. Silence is also okay.

"That's something I learned with my patient," Shyanne smiles. "Sometimes she's okay with silence; she just sits listening to the clock ticking or the cars going by outside. It's about giving someone the truth of who you are, and just being there. That's very difficult in our society because we equate *being* with *being unproductive*. For me, it's the truest sense of achievement. You can just hang out, give of yourself, and be in the moment.

"I don't know how old you are, but if you've taken this many years to get to where you are—doing, doing, doing—you're not going to suddenly be this incredible human *being* with a few weeks of exposure to hospice. So be gentle with yourself, accept that it's going to take a while, and be patient."

I know Shyanne is right. I recall my interview with Chris earlier in the day, and the realization that I need to worry less about entertaining Dorothy and learn how to just *be with* her. I'm working too hard and I need to "be a nonanxious presence," as Patrice said during the training. Although Dorothy has never said outright that I'm not doing what she needs, I want reassurance that she feels my visits are worthwhile for her.

Shyanne has adapted to even more extreme differences between herself and her patient, so I want to know how she interprets her role in her patient's life.

Shyanne thinks for a moment and then says, "She deals a lot with loneliness, and I know that she's wanted a volunteer since January but they had not been able to find one who was prepared to go into that neighborhood. After figuring out who I was and what I was about, we talked about politics and skin color and children and raising kids and husbands. She has a lot of views on George W. Bush and what he's going to do for the country and what he isn't going to do. She's a fascinating woman. For someone with an elementary school education she really has attended the school of life, I think, very well.

"I think she sees me as a friend and also as someone to maybe pass on some of her wisdom to. She taught me how to cook squash the other day. I thought I knew how to cook squash, but she told me I didn't. So, I went and bought some little yellow goose-necked squash and she instructed me. She's in a lot of pain, so she sat down on the chair in her little kitchen. There were roaches everywhere and rat droppings, it was very offensive—but I cooked squash! She instructed me step by step. And I'm a vegetarian and she had me putting tablespoons of pork fat in the squash. It was quite an experience," Shyanne laughs and then drops her voice, leaning forward almost conspiratorially, "And I *ate* it—and it tasted delicious!"

I observe, "It seems she has a sense of her legacy, these pearls of wisdom, wanting to teach you how to make squash so that her knowledge gets passed on."

Shyanne smiles and laughs. "And I'll never ever forget it! It'll be something that I'll remember when I'm 80 years old—me standing in her kitchen, cooking the squash, cooking the *life* out of the squash. As a vegetarian, I steam everything and then eat it immediately, and we were cooking stuff that looked like yellow snot!" Shyanne laughs again. "With pork fat in it! It was just the funniest experience, and it tasted heavenly."

"But probably not like squash at all."

"No! It took on a life of its own."

Just like these relationships with our patients, I think. Perhaps that's what I'm missing so far. I haven't relinquished enough control to allow our relationship to grow a life of its own. Later in the interview, Shyanne shares another observation that inspires me and gives me further insight into hospice relationships as growth and change.

Shyanne says passionately, "It's such a beautiful, growth place, such fertile ground—but you have to come to a place where there's no expectation. It's like throwing wildflower seeds out there—you have no idea what's going to grow—but also you start it with fallow ground that doesn't have anything in it. That's how I see us—as growing a garden together. We have gardening as a common interest. I have a beautiful flower garden here in my home. I live just 5 minutes down the street in a little old, 60-year-old restored house; it's really beautiful but I love the outside more than the inside. So she was asking, 'What's growing?' And I think that's symbolic. She says, 'What's growing today?' And I say, 'Well, my snapdragons came up.' So we talk about the colors of the snapdragons and how I need to feed them. And she's got all these things that I need to put on my garden that are not chemical based. 'You need to take the tea out of the tea bags and put it around the snapdragons,' she says.

"But to me, it's symbolic as to what else is going on in our lives. We're growing each other. Before, I was this beautiful strong tree with so much to offer, but I was straight up and down. Now, I'm growing all these interesting shoots and twigs and branches and they're not orderly and they're not in control and I don't give a darn. There's no symmetry and that's okay. Some of them have knots in them and some of them are not going to go anywhere, and that's okay. But I do try to keep that in mind. She's like a beautiful old tree to me."

I am mesmerized by Shyanne's vision of the tree, and amazed by her ability to weave a story, complete with imagery and metaphor. As we say our goodbyes and part company, I know that this interview is Shyanne's gift to me, and I can hardly wait to share it. I have one more interview to complete, with Hannah, and I think I will bring a renewed sense of optimism to my next visit with Dorothy.

HANNAH

On the evening of our graduation from hospice, Hannah raced into the meeting a few minutes late, having driven back across the bay after a long day working at the Attorney General's office in a neighboring county. Hannah is tall and slender, with long curly hair that she confesses she rarely has time to cut. I wonder how she finds time for hospice and what motivates her to do so. We meet on a Thursday evening at a coffee shop near the university. I feel uneasy that Hannah is driving out of her way to meet me on my home territory, but she assured me that it was no trouble for her. I soon discover that most of what Hannah does is motivated by an enormous generosity and empathy for other people. Within moments, I feel like I am chatting with an old girlfriend, and the tape of our interview is marked by the sounds of cooperative overlaps at the ends of sentences, resounding "yeahs" and "exactlys," and even finishing each other's thoughts.

As in all the interviews, I begin by asking Hannah how she became a hospice volunteer.

"Actually, it just happened by chance. I was in the mall one day, and they were having a service organization fair of some kind. I wasn't even intending to go to that section of the mall, I just happened to walk by there and I saw it. It just sort of struck me, and I filled out the paperwork. I'd never heard anything about it before. I was just about to graduate, and for 3 years, my every waking moment had been taken up with law school, so I didn't get to do anything. I consider myself pretty lucky, so after law school I wanted to do something to help someone else or somehow repay all the good fortune that I've had.

"There's one organization where you rebuild old houses and then somebody gets the house. To me, that's wonderful, but you don't see the family that gets it, so you don't see what you're doing for somebody else. In hospice, you see your patient each day that you visit them, you have that interaction with them, and it's such a good thing. So, when I saw the table and the lady just sitting there, I thought, 'This is what I'm going to do.' I filled out the paperwork and here I am. I had never heard of it before, not even in the nursing home where I volunteered."

I am surprised that Hannah has never heard of hospice, particularly when she tells me that 12 years earlier she and her mother took care of her grandmother until she died. That experience, combined with some time spent volunteering at a retirement home, drew her to hospice the first time she heard of it. I ask if there is anything else in her upbringing that might have prompted her to approach a volunteering booth during a trip to the mall.

Hannah responds thoughtfully, "I have two younger siblings and then an 8-year-old in the family. I'm 4 years older than my sister and 5 years older than my brother, and my parents worked very hard their whole lives, so I practically raised my siblings. Volunteering is a part of who I am—something that makes me happy. My brother and sister are now married and they have their own families. I don't, so I look for other ways to do something for someone—if that makes any sense."

We spend some time comparing notes on the training program, and agree that we covered a lot of material but neither of us felt totally prepared.

Hannah leans her head to one side a little as she reflects, "It was much more personal than I thought it would be. I think that's how you get people interested and how you get people wanting to stay. Because if a problem comes up, I can go to any one of them and they're going to be there to help me. It's an uncomfortable situation if you're out there alone, struggling, and you think that if you call they'll think you're stupid."

I confess. "I prefer situations where I know what I'm doing, and when it came to hospice, I was afraid of messing up. The training helped me to realize not only that there was very little I could do to mess up, but also that other people were a little nervous about it as well."

Like Tom, Chris, and Emilia, Hannah is volunteering in a nursing home and I ask her to describe her first visit with her patient.

"Well," Hannah begins, "I knew the basics, like what she likes to do and what her diagnosis is. Patrice said if we didn't get along then I could see someone else. But I knew right away that I would stick with it even before I met her, because Patrice told me that this woman had been married for 50-some-odd years, but she'd never had any kids and all her siblings had died. So, she was there all by herself. She had only one nephew who had his own family, and according to the paperwork, he couldn't go to see her that often. So, I knew I would keep her because her situation was what I was afraid of for myself—being by yourself and knowing that you were going to die.

"After I met her nephew I knew that he loved her a great deal, but she didn't have any kids, and she didn't have her husband, so she really did spend her days all alone. I knew right away that she could have been the worst patient ever and I would have taken her. It was exactly what I needed, which goes back to being in the right place at the right time—and fate.

"When I got there, she was actually very temperamental, but I thought it was interesting, and she was a lot better than I thought she would be—I mean, physically. She was very alert. She had lung cancer, or so they thought, but she wouldn't let them take a biopsy, so it was questionable, but that's what it appeared to be. She also had heart failure and she would run out of breath very quickly, but she didn't want me to stop talking. Well, you know I'm an attorney, and I talk a *lot*, and I thought it was comical that she didn't care what I said."

Hannah smiles and continues, "At one point, I was going to say goodnight because I noticed she was out of breath when she was talking back to me. And she said, 'No, don't leave.' And I said, 'Well, what do you want to talk about?' And she said, 'It doesn't matter to me, you can talk about anything you want, just keep talking.' So I did. She didn't talk back very much, but she was *so* glad for the company. She kept thanking me for stopping by and for just sitting with her, and I realized that she was a little bit happier. I was there for a little over an hour because she was getting too tired, but for that hour, I realized that at least she wasn't alone.

"And the nurse there," Hannah shakes her head. "My patient was in pain when I went, and she asked me to go to the nurse and get her something, and the nurse was just very mean to her. For whatever reason, my patient wanted to put her medicine on top of her little dinner table—but the nurse wouldn't let her. They kept going back and forth. Finally, my patient took the medicine and spoke really slowly to the nurse, as if she was a fifth grader: 'Now, wait a minute, before you take it back, I'm *just going to lay it here.*' And I just thought it was so funny!

"When the nurse finally left, my patient turns around to me and says, 'I'm glad you're here because you can see that it's not me. People think that I'm mean, but it's not me! It's *her!*' It was funny how even in light of everything that had happened to her—she knew she was passing—and yet she had a sense of humor about her situation."

"I wonder how she knew that other people thought she was mean," I ask. "Or perhaps she was just responding to the nurse's attitude toward her?"

"Perhaps the nurse was just having a bad day, but I also imagine that you get a little frustrated when you're older. Perhaps you were a much nicer person when you were younger and happier and you weren't sitting in a nursing home for 24 hours a day. I also think that the staff is not very kind. They forget that the patients are there all day long.

"For example," Hannah continues, "At one point my patient said, 'Well, my chest hurts.' And the nurse just stood there and said, 'Well, you know why that is? It's because you have heart failure. You *know* why this lady is here. You *know* she's from hospice.' So, if she hadn't spoken to her nephew that day and if I hadn't been there, that could've been her only interaction all day! How sad that would've been! At least she got to chit chat—or listen to me chit chat! Especially to someone in a nursing home, having someone kind to talk to makes a difference."

That was the first and only time Hannah got to spend time with her patient alone.

"I visited her on a Thursday, and I was going back the next week on Wednesday, and that morning Patrice called to tell me she had taken a turn for the worse and she was in the dying process, which was odd because I had just spoken to her and she was fine. I went back that night, and her nephew was there with his wife, and my patient didn't look right. You could tell that she was passing. I went over and she immediately knew who I was. She squeezed my hand and her nephew's wife said, 'Hannah's here,' and she said my name."

I am moved that Hannah's patient and the family members responded to her so warmly, welcoming her into that intimate scene even though Hannah had only visited her one time.

Hannah continues, "The next morning I got a call that she was even more alert than the night before, but then she passed away during that day. So it was not what I expected. Even hospice was surprised she was so alert, but they knew that she was dying. When you think of the dying process, you think of someone who's not speaking, not eating. The night I was there, she was still drinking water, so it was kind of strange. At least I got the chance to meet her nephew and his wife, which was nice."

With such a brief encounter, I am curious to know how Hannah had interpreted the meaning of her experience and her relationship to the patient.

"I don't think it's just the patient; I think it's the family, too. I only met my patient's nephew the second day I was there, but I immediately knew how grateful he was that she hadn't been by herself. When she said my name, I saw him smiling, and I thought, 'I'm sure that made him happy.' I stayed for an hour talking about all the things she'd told me, and they told me stories about her. It was an hour where she was dying but we laughed, and they laughed and they joked, and in my mind she heard all this and I think that it must have made her happy. As I left, I asked them to stop thanking me because I didn't really do anything. They thanked me profusely for sitting with her and for spending time with them."

I reflect, "It's about witnessing, like you say, witnessing at that time, and honoring whatever that experience is—saying, 'This is important, too.'"

"So, your patient's alert and doing fine?" Hannah inquires.

"Yeah! I visit her at home and, really, in a 2-hour visit, she may have one coughing spell. She's got oxygen, but that's the only outward sign.

She's frail but she's clearly never been a big lady. We're slowly getting to know each other, particularly this week, because we're making plans to go out together. I'm starting to get a sense of who I am to her. We don't talk about anything deep—like with your lady when she said, 'Just talk.'"

"Keep me company," Hannah adds.

"And you did, but you got a sense of what that meant to her. So I'm really happy that my relationship with Dorothy is developing. It's also scary to me, because I remember that the only reason I'm there is that at some point she's going to say goodbye—sooner rather than later. So, I wanted to ask you about being the witness for your patient but at the same time being able to separate. Knowing that it's not your own death, and it's not even the death of a relative, you've got to be sensitive but at the same time ...."

"I don't know how you do that," Hannah interjects. "Do you *want* to be able to distance yourself? If at the end of your visit you were like, 'Okay, well, that's it. Now I won't really think about it.' Are you doing anything for that person? I honestly don't think so. I feel you have to become a part of their lives to make their lives better. Their death has to move you; to somehow affect you. That's when you know you've done something wonderful. If their death meant something to you, then your being there meant something to them. I think that's why we do this."

I ask Hannah about her patient and whether hospice gave her the option to be there once her patient was in the dying process.

"Yeah, they did. They said that I should do whatever I felt comfortable with. If I wanted to go, great, and if I didn't they would understand. They were going to try to put a volunteer with her all day because she didn't want to die alone. I'm not 100% sure that somebody was there when she passed, but I do know that they tried to get volunteers to sit with her."

The idea of vigil volunteering interests me greatly. I observe, "Before the training, I assumed that hospice ensured that patients didn't die alone. But then in the training they said, 'That would be great if that could happen, but it's too difficult.' And I'd never thought about hospice in nursing homes, which is, I'm sure, where you're going to get people who are ...."

"By themselves?" Hannah suggests.

"Yeah, by themselves. I would love to see a world in which someone was there to note the passing of every human being."

"It's such a sad thing, isn't it?" Hannah shakes her head and looks down at her hands holding her coffee cup. "It really is. It frightens me a lot. I'm very young, and I hope not to pass for many, many years. But it's a scary thing, and it happens, I'm sure, every day."

"Would you be interested in doing that kind of vigil work for hospice?"

"I would," Hannah agrees, looking up at me again. "I think I would like it a lot. Unfortunately, there's so much I would like to do and work doesn't leave me with much time. But I did list that as one of my choices, as long as it was when I could go. If I had been able to get the time sit with my patient, I would have, but with court it's impossible for me to just get up and leave. Although I think it would be a little scary, to tell you the truth; it would be sad and a little frightening, but I would love to have the chance to do it.

"When you think about it, for somebody to share that, it is just an incredible thing. To have that opportunity to be the last person there as they said goodbye, I almost think of it as a privilege. I never thought about it like that until we did the hospice training and I realized—I always thought dying was sad. I really did."

Hannah seems to have had a condensed version of the hospice experience. She met with a patient and experienced a level of meaningful contact with her, including interacting with the family, and then said goodbye. Given the short length of the average stay in hospice, I am reassured that Hannah was able to fulfill her role as a volunteer in a short space of time, and walk away feeling that she made a difference to her patient and her patient's family. Although she spoke about a patient's death needing to move us in some way, I also note that Hannah appears to have taken the death of her patient in stride, which is how it is supposed to be when we volunteer for hospice. At the same time, I wonder what it is like to lose a patient after visiting her or him for several weeks or months. I suspect it is harder to achieve a sense of meaningful closure and acceptance. I have been visiting Dorothy for a month now, and I am not yet sure of what, if anything, I contribute to her quality of life. Although she can no longer drive and is a terminal hospice patient, Dorothy appears quite self-sufficient and I wonder to what extent she even needs a volunteer. I'm not sure how I would feel if she suddenly "took a turn for the worse," except that I wouldn't be sure that I had helped her in any way.

Perhaps Shyanne is right when she says that I am too judgmental about the whole situation, and maybe it is enough just to be there. Chris said essentially the same thing when he made the analogy between the tree falling in the forest and the life that is isolated without human contact. Maybe I don't need to make certain things happen between Dorothy and me, or make this relationship fit into a familiar category, such as friend, or family, or even patient. One thing that I've learned from these first interviews is that there is no cookie-cutter answer to the challenges I face with Dorothy, and that's what makes this experience so valuable to me. Discovering what Dorothy needs and responding to her uniqueness as an individual may be all I need to do to fulfill what hospice intends with its philosophy of person-centered care. However, like so many other theories regarding human interaction— such as dialogue, or invitational rhetoric, or unconditional positive regard—it is an idea that looks easy on paper but is deceptively complicated in practice. When all's said and done, I can spend as much time as I want planning my responses to Dorothy in my mind, but it is meaningless until I actually surrender enough control and judgment to experience being with her. Perhaps our outings will allow us to focus on something *together,* rather than feeling compelled to engage in question and answer sessions. I suppose I will find out when I next visit Dorothy in a few days.

5

Going Out

THE FISHING PIER

After I had mentally prepared myself to take Dorothy out for a drive 2 weeks ago, Terry's older daughter, Sharon, came in from out of town to visit Dorothy, so we stayed at home with her. Dorothy and I did discuss some ideas about where to go, and Dorothy decided she would like to drive to the fishing pier where she and Stan used to fish. I was glad to find that it is not too far away and I actually know how to get there. But our outing was postponed again the following week when, at the last minute, Dorothy's nurse, Jackie, had to change her appointment and it coincided with my visit. Dorothy did not seem concerned, so I didn't worry about it either.

I called Dorothy last night to make sure she still felt well enough to go.

"Don't you worry about me," Dorothy said, happily. "I'm as fit as a fiddle!"

Today, after receiving instructions from Terry about how to manage the portable oxygen tank, Dorothy and I finally drive down to the fishing pier. I take a route that brings us along Bayshore Boulevard, with the sparkling bay on our left and million dollar homes on our right. I feel relaxed sitting in silence as we drive because I can see that Dorothy is enjoying the view.

We pull up under a tree in a parking space that is close to the pier and only a short walk to a picnic table with an unobstructed view of the bay and the city skyline.

Before we get out, I ask Dorothy, "Would you like to walk out to the pier or sit at the table for a while?"

"We could take a walk," Dorothy replies. "I don't think I want to take this oxygen, though, I really don't need it."

"Are you sure? I wouldn't want you to get tired out."

"I won't get tired," Dorothy says, emphatically. Then she adds, "If I do, we can just sit down or get back in the car."

"Okay," I agree. I'm nervous about Dorothy walking around out here without her oxygen, but I can't insist that she wear it if she doesn't want to. I wonder if she feels self-conscious about wearing the oxygen out in public. I can certainly understand if she does.

We walk out onto the pier and look over the railings into the water. We've arrived at low tide and the water is so clear that we can see down to the stones and sand around the pier. I stay close to Dorothy in case she needs a hand with the steps or negotiating the uneven, wooden boards of the pier, but she doesn't seem to need my help. I ask about her fishing trips and she tells me that she and Stan used to come here at night, and they would usually catch something.

"There's usually a lot more people here at night," Dorothy says. "And a lot more fish, too," she adds.

"I don't see any fish here now," I comment.

"Nope," Dorothy says, "me neither. We'd be going home hungry if we were fishing today."

"Did you cook the fish you caught, Dorothy?" I ask.

"Yes," Dorothy says, "we cooked it. Or, I should say, Stan cooked it. I never did the cooking in my house. But I sure know how to cook fish. I made the best catfish and hushpuppies in Alabama."

"I love catfish," I say. "Never had it until I moved to Memphis when I was 24."

"You were missing out then!" Dorothy exclaims. "Don't they have catfish where you're from?"

I think about it for a moment and then reply, "You know what, Dorothy? I really don't know if they have catfish there or not. I'd heard of a catfish before I moved to Memphis, but I never ate one."

"They're good, aren't they?!" Dorothy says, smiling.

"They sure are." I return her smile.

It's starting to get very warm out on the pier and we've been standing for a while. "Do you want to go sit down at the picnic table?" I ask.

"We can do that if you want to." Dorothy turns to walk back slowly along the pier.

I'm becoming accustomed to Dorothy's standard reply of "if you want to." She has yet to disagree with anything I suggest, so I must trust my instincts. I would feel a lot better if Dorothy took the lead and told me what she needs, but perhaps that's just not her style. The main concern I have is that we will repeat what happened with the checkers game—she will agree to do something that she doesn't want to do, just because she thinks it's what I want. I also know that I am feeling but not saying a lot of things in the interest of maintaining the tenuous connections we've made so far. Perhaps Dorothy is just doing the same thing—which means she is trying to make this work, too; I try to stop myself from analyzing every sign and nuance that would help me know how things are going between Dorothy and me.

We sit on the same side of the picnic table, looking out over the water. It is a beautiful day and the silences in our conversation don't seem to bother me as much while we have this view to occupy us. Dorothy seems relaxed, too, and that helps me to worry less about entertaining her. We chat intermittently about places that Dorothy has lived, and at one point, I see a group of dolphins surface out in the bay.

"Look, Dorothy!" I exclaim, "Did you see the dolphins?"

"No," she replies, "Where are they?"

"They're about 200 yards straight out, and they're heading toward our left," I reply. "I'm sure they'll come up again in a moment."

Dorothy's eyes scan the water and, just when I think they're gone, they surface.

Dorothy exclaims, "Look! There they are!" Six or seven of the unmistakable dorsal fins arch out of the water and disappear again.

After a few moments of silence, I say, "I love dolphins."

"I do, too," Dorothy agrees.

We sit for a little while and wait for the dolphins to resurface, but we don't see them again. As we stand to walk back to the car, I look down and see a large ant on Dorothy's arm.

"Dorothy, there's an ant …." I don't finish the thought, but grasp the tiny offender and throw it to the ground. For a moment, I am surprised by how intimate this gesture feels to me, probably because of the protective instinct that prompted it.

"Thank you, honey," Dorothy says. "He could've given me quite a pinch."

"You're right," I reply. "Those bites can sting for ages."

As I help Dorothy into the car, she says, "Maybe I should wear my oxygen on the way home."

"Do you need help?" I ask.

"No, I've got it," she replies, pulling the tubes and nasal cannula out from the carrying case, and hooking them over her ears.

I close her door and smile as I walk to the driver's side.

It's getting easier, I think.

DOROTHY'S RESTAURANT

During my regular Monday night calls to Dorothy, I always say, "I'll see you tomorrow at 10 o'clock," so that she knows when to expect me. Recently, I noticed that Dorothy has begun to reply, 'Ten or 10:30. It doesn't matter. Whatever is best for you.'

I now decode Dorothy's indirect communication style and recognize that 10:30 must be a better time for her, so I make my visits a little later than I originally planned.

As I walk toward Dorothy's apartment, I see that Terry has arranged a few chairs and a small table in the breezeway. I am surprised to see a filled ashtray and I wonder briefly who has been smoking.

Terry's husband, Len, answers the door. I recognize him immediately from the photographs I have seen around the house. Although I learned from Dorothy that Len stays at the apartment every other weekend, this is the first time we've met.

I hold out my hand, "Hi, I'm Elissa. I'm Dorothy's volunteer."

"Len Holmes," he says, shaking my hand a little awkwardly and looking toward the ground, "Terry's husband."

"Yes," I reply. "I recognize you from the photos. Pleased to meet you."

As I enter the living room, Dorothy announces, "Terry! The babysitter's here!"

As usual, Dorothy is sitting in her chair wearing her oxygen. A reality courtroom program plays on the television, the blinds are drawn, and the lamps are lit. I find it comforting that things tend to stay the same around here.

"How are you doing, Dorothy?" I smile and move to my spot on the sofa near Dorothy.

"I'm fine. How are you?" Dorothy asks with a smile.

"I'm fine. Working hard," I reply.

"I know you are," Dorothy says. "Those kids at the school not giving you too much trouble, I hope."

"Not too much," I reply. This exchange is a regular ritual now.

"Have you met Len?" Dorothy asks.

"We just met at the door," I reply. "How are you doing, Len? I've heard a lot about you."

"All bad, of course," Dorothy teases.

"I've heard a lot about you, too," Len says. He hovers near the doorway and I realize that I've made myself at home in my usual spot on the sofa while Len seems uncomfortable. I wonder if I should have waited for Len to invite me in, but Dorothy seems happy, so I relax and decide not to worry about it. Len's coloring is as dark as Terry's is fair, but he is about the same height as she is. His build is quite strong and heavy; his shoulders are broad and his chest and midsection are thick. Then, I notice that his forearms and legs are surprisingly slender, which reminds me that he sits for hours and hours every day behind the wheel of his truck.

Terry walks into the living room from the hallway. "Hi, how are you doing?" she asks with a broad smile. "Did you meet Len?"

"Yes, thank you," I reply.

"He's been driving long trips up the East Coast for a couple of months, so he's taking a week off," Terry explains.

"Sounds like hard work," I say to Len.

"It's not too bad," Len replies, still avoiding eye contact with me. "I'm used to it."

I remember the cigarettes on the table outside and realize that Len must be the smoker; perhaps that's why he's hovering near the door.

"I'm just about to make another pot of coffee, would you like some?" Terry asks.

"No, thank you," I reply.

"Len?" she asks.

"Yeah, thanks," Len replies, then turns to address me. "Excuse me; I'm just going to step outside for a minute."

Once Len has closed the door, Terry confirms, "He's gone outside to have a cigarette, you know. I don't think he should be smoking in the house any more."

Dorothy interjects, "Well, it doesn't bother me, and it's *my* place. Smoking never bothered me," Dorothy turns to address me, "Some people don't like it after they give up smoking, they don't want it around them, but it never bothered me. I smoked for 60-odd years, and gave up cold turkey."

I nod silently, but say nothing.

"That's great, Mom," Terry says, firmly, "but Len doesn't need to be smoking inside; he can sit out there and be quite comfortable. Now, would you like some coffee, Mom?" It's clear that Terry means this to be the final word.

"No thanks," Dorothy replies, "I think I'll wait until we go to the restaurant."

I catch Terry shaking her head as she walks to the kitchen.

Dorothy leans over and confides to me, "I don't mind Len smoking in the house. I think it's mean of her to make him go outside all by himself to smoke. It's my place and I don't care about him smoking. You know what I'm saying?"

"I think so," I reply. "Maybe Terry is just worried about having the smoke around you because you're on the oxygen?"

"She doesn't have to worry about me!" Dorothy says, indignantly. "I can speak for myself!"

I immediately realize my faux pas and try to amend it. "Maybe Terry doesn't like having smoke in the house because she doesn't smoke."

Dorothy nods, "Well, that may be true, too."

Terry walks through the living room to take a cup of coffee to Len, and then joins us in the living room. We talk for a little while about

Terry's daughters and events in the lives of other relatives. After a few minutes, Dorothy rises from her chair.

"I have to go to the bathroom," she says. "Then would you like to get a bite to eat?" she asks me.

"Sure," I reply, "as soon as you're ready."

"Alright then!" Dorothy says as she walks down the hallway, holding her oxygen line. "Got to remember to take my tail with me."

I love Dorothy's little joke, which she makes about once every visit. Terry sinks back into her chair and exhales audibly—a weary sigh.

"How are you doing, Terry?" I ask.

"I'm fine, a little tired I guess," she replies taking a sip of her coffee. "I've been picking up some work through this temp agency down on the corner. The extra money's good to have, but I'm worth a lot more than they pay me. I'm not always sure it's worth it."

"I didn't know you were doing that," I say. "I've done some temp work before. It's true the agencies charge a lot of money for you, compared to what they pay."

"Yeah, well," Terry replies. "I don't have too many options. I can't take anything regular because of Mom, but we really do need some extra money coming in."

I nod silently. This is the first I've heard about the finances of Dorothy and Terry's household, but it makes sense that they would be struggling a little, particularly if Terry is usually employed full-time.

"Yeah," Terry continues. "I've been a teller for 16 years, ever since my youngest went to school. The banks are getting rid of a lot of those positions, though, so I'm not even sure I'll be able to get something permanent after I stop taking care of Mom. You know how you're not supposed to accept full-time work from someone you temp for without telling the agency? Well, they can shove it! I'd accept a position in a heartbeat and never tell them anything."

I think that it must have been difficult for Terry to uproot her life and move to take care of Dorothy, but I'm glad she did. In temperament, Terry reminds me of my grandmother—strong, stoic, friendly but not overtly affectionate, with a tendency to demonstrate her love through actions rather than words. I predict that Terry's comment about the temp agency is the closest I'll ever come to hearing her complain about anything.

Dorothy walks slowly back into the living room. "Are you ready to go?" she asks me.

"Sure," I reply, "Where would you like to go today?"

"Do you know the Crossroads Diner?" Dorothy asks. "It's down on Broad Street."

"I'm afraid I don't know that area of town, Dorothy," I reply.

"Wow," Terry exclaims, "the old Crossroads Diner! What made you think of that place, Mom?"

"Well," Dorothy says, "We never go down there any more, and it's a good restaurant!"

Terry explains, "It's in the old neighborhood, where Mom and Dad used to live."

"Great! Do you remember the way, Dorothy?" I ask.

"Sure do," Dorothy replies. "I used to drive all over this town."

As we leave, we pass Len sitting in the breezeway. He has a newspaper, which I guess he must have picked up from the machine near the rental office, and he is quietly reading with his coffee and his cigarette. He looks comfortable and I tell him so.

Len smiles, shyly, "It's nice to have a little time to read the paper."

"I'm sure it is," I respond, hoping to draw him out a bit.

"Maybe we'll see you later?" he says, looking directly at me for the first time.

"We're going to the Crossroads," Dorothy says as if to move the conversation along. I can tell she's eager to get on the road, and that makes me feel good.

"Have fun," Len replies.

We drive down to Dorothy's old neighborhood and I see the Crossroads Diner for the first time. It is a single-story brick building, which, I am certain, has not changed for 20 years. Even before we push open the front door, I note the handwritten sign that says, "No cards." I wonder if this is because it costs more money to handle credit cards, or whether they simply prefer the old way of doing things. Inside the diner is a counter with a row of six stools extending most of the way across the small building, with a cash register at one end and the kitchen immediately behind. Three waitresses stride briskly through the space behind the counter, pouring coffee and passing their orders back to the kitchen. The rest of the seating consists of about 14 booths arranged in an L shape along two sides of the building. Each booth is big enough to seat two people comfortably or possibly three, but only if two are very thin and don't mind sitting close together.

As we pause to look for a seat, one of the waitresses calls out, "Smoking in the front, nonsmoking in the back."

Because the booths run in an L, there is no physical separation between smoking and nonsmoking, and I am surprised that the diner is considered big enough to have a designated smoking section.

Dorothy claims a booth in the front despite the other patrons who are smoking nearby. It bothers me, but I don't say anything.

A petite, dark-haired waitress walks up to the booth with two menus and two glasses of water, which she places in front of us.

"The soup today is baked potato or beef and vegetable," she says, then pulls a pen from behind her ear with one hand and a pad from her back pocket with another. "What can I get you to drink today?"

"I'll have a cup of coffee," Dorothy says. She points to the glass of water, "But you can take that away. It'll rust my insides."

"I'll have a coffee, too," I add. "But I'll keep the water if you don't mind."

"So, do you remember me?" Dorothy looks up at the waitress expectantly.

"'Course I do, Dorothy," the waitress responds, smiling. "We haven't seen you around here lately. How're you doing?"

"I'm doing fine," she says, then nods in my direction. "This is my friend. We eat lunch together."

"Pleased to meet you." Turning from the table, she says, "I'll get that coffee for you."

Dorothy smiles and tells me that she and Stan used to come here every night for dinner.

"The house we had is just around the corner, and we would drive over here, sometimes we'd walk, but mostly we'd drive. And we got to know these girls pretty well. That one who waited on us is Debbie."

I smile at Dorothy's use of the word *girls*. Debbie appears to be the youngest of the three waitresses, and she is certainly over 40. It occurs to me that anyone younger than Dorothy's daughters must seem like girls to her.

"Maybe I could show you my house some time," Dorothy suggests. She points to the menu. "Take a look at the menu. See what you'd like. They generally have good food here."

I scan the laminated menu and soon realize that ordering will be easy because I don't eat beef, pork, or chicken. I choose the fish sandwich; Dorothy decides on a ham and cheese omelet.

When Debbie returns with our coffee, we are ready to order. I notice Dorothy looking around the diner, I assume for faces that she recognizes.

"When were you last here?" I ask.

"I think it was a year ago, maybe longer. It was after I moved to that apartment, but I still had my car. I came down here with someone ...." Her voice trails off as she drifts into memory.

I look around the diner, too. Many of our fellow patrons appear to be employees of the neighborhood businesses—two women in medical uniforms, a mechanic, two men with pest control logos on their shirts, and two male police officers. I wonder if they are regulars.

"Did you come here alone after Stan passed away?" I ask.

"Yes. For a long time I used to come here by myself, or with one of the girls when they came to visit. Sometimes I would sit with a friend."

Dorothy smiles and takes a sip of her coffee.

"A friend from the neighborhood?"

"Yes. He lived in the apartments just behind the restaurant. We used to see each other, you know, just to say hello. Sometimes he had dinner with his grandson, but mostly he ate alone, like me. One day there were no booths when he came and I said, 'Do you want to share a booth?' because I was alone and he was alone. It didn't make sense for him to wait for a seat."

"Right," I agree. "And so you started having dinner together?"

"Every night." Dorothy smiles, wistfully.

An idea forms and I decide to take a risk. I wouldn't normally ask such a direct question, but I really want to know. "Dorothy," I pause for a moment, "did you have a *boyfriend*?"

Dorothy chuckles, "Well, it wasn't a sexual thing, if that's what you mean!"

"Dorothy!" I exclaim and burst into laughter. Given my own tentativeness about asking a personal question, Dorothy's openness catches me off guard. I am simultaneously surprised and delighted. Perhaps the restaurant has put her at ease, but I prefer to think that we are finally getting to know each other. I continue to smile and look at Dorothy expectantly.

Dorothy grins in response to my reaction. "He was a good friend." After a moment, Dorothy's mischievous expression changes to one of sadness as she looks down at her coffee.

"What happened?" I ask quietly, already suspecting the answer.

"He died," Dorothy replies, simply. "He just died one day. They said it was a stroke. His daughter came down to the restaurant to tell me."

I feel terrible. "I'm very sorry, Dorothy. It sounds like you two got to be close."

"We did," Dorothy nods looking down at the coffee mug in her hands. Then she looks up and smiles. "But you know what? When The Man Upstairs calls your number, there's nothing you can do. Don and I had some good times together, but then it was time for him to go."

"I guess you're right."

Debbie walks up to the table with our lunch. "Here you go. Ham and cheese omelet, fish sandwich, and your fries will be up in a second, Hon," she says to me.

"How about some more coffee, here?" Dorothy orders gruffly, faking a frown.

"You always were a bossy old thing, Dorothy," Debbie says, winking at me.

After Debbie walks away from the table, Dorothy leans toward me across the table, as if to reassure me, "She and I always kid around like that."

I smile as we both pick up our cutlery and begin our lunch.

As we sit and eat in silence, I look around the Crossroads Diner again. This time, I can see why Dorothy loves it so much. I'm grateful that so little has changed about the place and Dorothy can come here and feel like she's home.

REFLECTIONS: SURMOUNTING THE STIGMA OF DYING

I am indebted to Henry, one of the volunteers who took part in two interviews in my study, who responded to the indeterminacy of dying with a thought-provoking phrase. When I spoke to Henry 6 months into volunteering, I confessed that I was having difficulty facing the inevitability of Dorothy's death. Henry replied that being with someone who was dying did not bother him. He said, "The way I see it, we're all dying, and this person [the patient] just happens to be a bit closer to it than I am." By reminding himself that he and his patients were equally mortal, he neutralized the negative connotations of dying, along with the inhibiting effects that the idea of death tends to have on conversations and relationships.

Compared to Henry, initially I found it difficult to put death and dying to the back of my mind when I thought about visiting patients. For some of the volunteers, their patient's disease and dying was, as Shyanne later expressed it, "a distant relative in the background," and for some it continued to influence our communication more directly. However, regardless of our sensitivity and consciousness about it, for all of us, death was an integral and inescapable element of the volunteer–patient relationship in hospice. Our very presence in our patients' lives depended entirely on the fact that they were dying, and our decision to become hospice volunteers meant that we were willing to face this fact, even if it meant confronting one of our deepest fears.

When I first considered volunteering for hospice, I believed that experiencing the death of a patient was the most effective way for me to address my fears about death and dying, and consequently learn how to communicate better in that context. Shyanne also came to hospice with the idea that volunteering would help her come to terms with this profound and inevitable aspect of existence. Shyanne's fear came from a childhood in which death was actively concealed from her and never discussed. Although death was never hidden from me as a child, I recall being afraid of death from an early age and my fear became a profound obstacle in my communication with my grandmother, and also my great aunt, when each of them was dying. At around the same time that my grandmother had lymphoma, I resisted visiting my great aunt who was living in a nursing home. Just thinking about it would make me suddenly hyper-conscious of her dying, and simultaneously, anxious to avoid any acknowledgment of her frailty, or my feelings. This same anxiety arose in me when I thought about talking with my grandmother explicitly about her illness. The paralysis I experienced appears to be a common reaction to dying as a culturally stigmatized state.

Goffman (1986) defines the stigmatized person as someone "possessing an attribute that makes him [sic] different from others in the category of persons available for him to be, and of a less desirable kind .... He is reduced in our minds from a whole and usual person to a tainted and discounted one" (pp. 2–3). In the end-of-life context, this means that once people's lives are punctuated by the judgment that they are dying, they are defined as *inherently* different from us rather than, as Henry perceived it, simply further along on the same journey. As Sontag (1990) points out, we all may hold dual citizenship but we identify ourselves as citizens of "that other place ... the kingdom of the ill," (p. 3) with great reluctance. My feelings about death caused me to see my relatives as different from me and different from the people they had been up to that point in time. In turn, this change in my perception caused me to distance myself from them, and made intimate communication with them extremely difficult. In my relationship with my grandmother, the stigmatizing effects of dying began as soon as my doctor told me the prognosis for a 70-year-old patient with lymphoma. Although I witnessed very few signs of my grandmother's deteriorating health, whenever I was in her presence, my mind became preoccupied with images of her approaching death—and these images frightened me. The awesome power of death—the fact that *I* could *be* and then *not be*—had intimidated me from an early age, and then my fears about mortality in a general sense became fixed upon my grandmother in a very personal sense.

Of course, the stigmatizing effects of death can be even worse when one is confronted by signs of physical frailty and declining health. Lawton (2000) conducted an extended study of patients at a residential hospice in England. "Patients repeatedly complained that other people had ceased both to see them and treat them as 'normal', particularly when the progression of their disease (or its treatment) affected their physical appearance" (Lawton, 2000, p. 44). Illustrating this phenomenon from the other side of the interaction, Kübler-Ross (1986) offers an account written by a student from one of her workshops whose close friend was dying of cancer:

> I called on him at home regularly in the months and weeks that followed, and gradually the truth started to sink in. He became thinner and weaker and finally was confined to a bed, a skeleton with white hair. I could not take it anymore and left. I never again saw him alive. He died several

weeks later .... And I guess I have never forgiven myself for deserting him during those last weeks. (p. xvi)

This story feels painfully familiar to me. When I knew that my grand-mother and great aunt needed support, I became emotionally over-whelmed and avoided facing my feelings. Despite caring a great deal about them and my relationships with them, I became preoccupied with their dying instead of responding to their living. My fear and antici-pated grief distracted me from my desire to be there and fueled my de-sire to escape the reality of their deaths.

In an ethnographic short story, Ellis (1995b) provides a vivid descrip-tion of her emotions during a conversation with her friend, Peter, who is dying of AIDS. In many ways, Ellis's account of her struggle to commu-nicate with her friend is made more poignant because she had already witnessed the death of her partner, Gene, some years before. "I can do this, I've done it many times. Talked of death, dying. I know what to say" (Ellis, 1995b, p. 77). Despite this insider knowledge of what it is like to be with someone who is dying, Ellis's attention remained locked on the physical signs of AIDS in Peter's body and on death—not a univer-sal and intangible death, but death at its most specific and intimate. In her reflections at the conclusion of the story, Ellis engaged the sense-making metaphor of being a visitor in the world of a dying per-son. She evaluated her encounter with her friend as "riddled with intersubjective failure" and asked, "Is it ever possible to connect the world of the living with the world of the dying?" (Ellis, 1995b, p. 81). As Ellis's story demonstrates, our visceral responses to the deterioration of the body constitute a significant obstacle to making this connection be-tween living and dying.

Our use of language can also constitute an obstacle in connecting the world of the living with the world of the dying; specifically, our atti-tudes and perceptions are distorted when we treat dying as a label and attach it to the person with whom we are trying to connect. Rather than recognizing and communicating with a person we care about who also happens to be dying, we fail to identify and defuse the effects of stigma-tization and instead communicate with a "dying person." Thus, we per-mit ourselves to privilege and respond to the fact they are dying and overlook the fact they—like us—are also living. We employ dying as a label that qualifies and diminishes their humanity, separating our-selves from them and constructing obstacles to communication that are similar to those we face with strangers. As defined by Gudykunst and Kim (1984):

Strangers represent both the idea of nearness in that they are physically close and the idea of remoteness in that they have different values and ways of doing things. Strangers are physically present and participating in a situation and at the same time are outside the situation because they are from a different place. (p. 20)

Communication with strangers is characterized by the "absence of familiar social scripts" (Gudykunst & Kim, 1984, p. 23) and a high degree of uncertainty associated with initial interaction (Berger & Calabrese, 1975). The effect of our construction of dying is a mirror image of this equation. The absence of a familiar social script for conversations about death and the high degree of uncertainty related to dying can cause us to treat even a close friend or relative who is dying as if he or she is a stranger.

As I mentioned in the introduction to Part II, although it can be helpful to think about the body as territory (Frank, 1991) or illness as a country (Ellis, 1995b; Morris, 1998; Sontag, 1990), it is important to remember that we all hold "dual citizenship" (Sontag, 1990, p. 3). This metaphorical adjustment implies that we can defuse stigmatization, not by ignoring or denying the significance of approaching death and what that means to the dying person, but by recognizing the duality of dying. *A dying person is also a living person.* The philosophy of hospice, the writings of Elisabeth Kübler-Ross (1986), and the revivalist movement (Seale, 1996; Walter, 1994) in general, emphasize the notion of "living until death." At a philosophical level, this re-visioning of dying implies that death is "not only a biological event but also an occasion, despite its sadness, suffused with positive cultural values and meanings" (Morris, 1998, p. 240). At an interpersonal level, this re-visioning implies overcoming the stigmatizing effects of both the physical signs of dying and dying as a label, in order to communicate in ways that validate and honor the life of the person and our relationship with him or her.

Beyond the effects of stigmatization, there is also the very tangible experience of fearing the impact of losing someone to death. When I asked Shyanne about her patient and if she ever worried about this in their relationship, she responded by reminding me of the principle of simply being there for our patients:

> I try really hard to be in the moment, because in order for me to be good in my profession, I have to walk my talk. And part of my talk is living in the moment and really appreciating where you are and not investing too much in tomorrow …. There's a certain boundary that I reserve for my own sanity, because I know that she will die eventually. And she knows that she will die. She doesn't like to talk about it very much. I don't know if that boundary will break down the more time I spend with her, but either way it will be a loss. I don't know how I'll react. I don't know how I'll feel until it happens.

Close friends and family members may not be able to establish boundaries in the same way that hospice volunteers can, particularly the caregivers who must constantly respond to the demands of an "unbounded" (Lawton, 2000) dying body. The strategy of focusing on the present is only one of many ways in which the volunteer experience diverges sharply from that of the caregiver. However, there may be momentary opportunities for family and friends to subdue consciously the anxiety that comes with thinking about the future and allow themselves to return to the present moment with loved ones who are dying. As difficult as it is to resist thinking about and anticipating what it will feel like to say goodbye, there is a huge cost if we focus only on the ending. As I did with my grandmother and great aunt, we risk missing the time we have to be with someone in the present, even if being with them means simply sitting in silence, wheeling them around a nursing home hallway, or cooking squash.

PART III

Communication as Improvisation: Learning How to"Be There" for People at the End of Life

Having taken the first steps with our hospice patients, and having es-chewed many of the myths and much of the initial uncertainty of be-coming volunteers, we began to establish our own level of comfort with the process of visiting and being with our patients. For those of us who continued to see the same patient for many months, our relationships developed to a point of connection and friendship even as we continued to learn about the boundaries and limitations of our role as hospice vol-unteers. Unlike in Part II, in which the interview stories were presented in a chapter separate from my stories of visiting Dorothy, Part III is orga-nized to illustrate three challenges that emerged once we had been vol-unteering for about 6 months: understanding our role in relation to both the living and the dying process of our patients—both as individuals and as members of hospice, learning to act as interpreters and media-tors for our patients who were not able to speak, and finding the balance between connecting to our patients and letting them go. In all three chapters of Part III, the stories are connected by the theme of improvisa-tion as the volunteers learned to respond in the moment and from our hearts while maintaining a sense of our hospice role.

Chapter 6 presents stories that reflect the challenge of finding our place within the lives of our patients as well as within the hospice orga-nization. A particular challenge that we did not anticipate is the possi-bility that our patients might not be dying in terms of the Medicare or hospice definition; thus, a question arises regarding the role of the hos-pice volunteer. If it is not to provide support as they are dying, what are we supposed to provide for our patients? In this respect, Chapter 6 deals primarily with issues of framing and sense making, and of identifying the boundaries of the hospice volunteer role. More concerned with the practices of volunteering, chapter 7 describes challenges of being with patients who cannot communicate through language or whose ability to hold a conversation is compromised. The stories in this chapter highlight the tendency within our culture to assume conversation to be *the* method through which relationships are established and maintained. This bias means that the volunteers had no scripts or cultural knowledge to help them know what to do when a patient could not (or would not) speak, and so they improvised. Chapter 8 tackles challenges related to interpersonal boundaries and the question of how closely we should connect with our patients in order to remain helpful and supportive as volunteers. In these stories in particular, but also throughout Part III, the volunteers discover what may be the quintessential balancing act (or dialectic) for all who face the challenges of communication at the end of life; namely, the balance between holding on and letting go.

Improvisation implies more than simply making things up as one goes along or "flying by the seat of one's pants." When used to describe interaction— whether between actors, athletes, musicians, or hospice volunteers and patients—improvisation implies a style of listening that is predicated on being fully present to the other person *and* being ready to respond meaningfully in the moment. Successful improvisation is also predicated on confidence in one's ability to perform as well as trust in the other person, both of which can be easier to achieve with the benefit of relationship history and experience. Conversely, Eisenberg (1990) described *jamming* as a mode of communication characterized by coordinated action, rather than shared meaning. He argued that too much relationship history can be an obstacle to the surrender of control that is required for improvisation. In the volunteers' interactions with patients, our confidence in ourselves and our relationships emerged over the first 6 months of volunteering, and although there is still evidence of uncertainty and nervousness in the stories that follow, there is also evidence that we are learning how to be there for our patients and their families.

6

Living in the Moment
Between Life and Death

THE COFFEE MAKER

Dorothy's granddaughter Leslie is staying with Terry and Dorothy again, as she was when I first came to visit at the beginning of the year. Dorothy has confided in me that Leslie's husband is "mean to her," which is why she comes to stay at the apartment sometimes. Although I am curious to know more about the situation, particularly if it is causing stress for Dorothy, I limit my questions to asking Dorothy how she feels about the situation. Although Dorothy feels bad about Leslie's predicament, I can tell that she is proud to be able to help Leslie by providing a place to stay. "Plenty of room for anyone who needs it," Dorothy tells me.

When I arrive this morning, Dorothy is alone. She informs me that Terry has a taken job for the day, and she doesn't know where Leslie is. Dorothy is sitting in her chair but is not wearing her oxygen. This does not immediately concern me, because I know that she has begun to leave it off for a few hours each day. Still, I sense that something is not quite right. I attribute my slight discomfort to the fact that Terry is not here.

"I haven't had my coffee this morning," Dorothy says, sounding frustrated.

"Why is that?"

"The coffee machine broke, the damn fool thing!" she exclaims. "I can't work out what's wrong with it."

"Would you like me to take a look?" I offer.

Dorothy waves her arm in the direction of the kitchen. "I don't know what you can do that I haven't tried already."

"Could you show me what you were doing? Sometimes all it takes is for someone else to take a look and it kind of fixes itself," I suggest.

"Well, do you want some coffee?" Dorothy asks.

"Yes, if we can get it going," I reply. I'm pretty sure Dorothy would not agree to let me fix the coffee machine if it was just for her sake.

Dorothy slowly rises from her chair and shuffles toward the kitchen. I follow her and watch what she does.

"Here's the problem," Dorothy points to the plastic basket that holds the coffee filter and grounds. It is sitting on the counter beside the coffee machine. "It won't go back in there." I watch Dorothy pick up the basket and try to maneuver it into place. She struggles, unsuccessfully, to fit the tiny hinge together and close the basket into place.

"See?" she says, "It's broken."

"Would you mind if I try?" I ask.

"Go ahead," Dorothy replies.

I take the basket back out from the precarious position in which Dorothy has left it, half in its hinge, half resting on top of the coffee pot. I slowly fit the top of the basket hinge into its slot, then click the bottom part into place, and swing it shut.

"Could you check to see if that's right?" I ask Dorothy.

Dorothy stretches her frail hands around the basket and wiggles it a little to test that it is securely in place.

"Well, that looks right to me," Dorothy says, sounding a little disquieted.

I'm afraid that she might feel embarrassed about not being able to repair her coffee maker, but rather than ask her about her feelings, I respond by acting as if everything is normal. "Shall we turn it on?" I ask.

"Sure," Dorothy replies, "we can do that. The button is right here." She pushes a small button on the bottom of the machine and the light goes on. Within a few seconds, we can hear the water starting to heat.

This is the first sign I've witnessed that Dorothy's condition is affecting her daily activities. Although this seems to be a very simple and quite harmless incident, I don't like it. I can tell that Dorothy is distressed, and I wonder if Terry has noticed Dorothy becoming confused in other ways. I'm concerned, but I don't know how to talk to Dorothy about it.

"Why don't we sit and watch some of *Texas Justice* while we wait for the coffee?" I suggest.

"Sure, we can do that, if you want," Dorothy replies.

When she gets to her chair, I pick up her oxygen tubes and say, "Would you like this, Dorothy? I can go and turn on the machine for you."

Dorothy waves the oxygen away with one hand and reaches for the remote control with the other. "I don't need it," she says. "I'm fine without it for a few hours. I don't want to become dependent on it, you know."

I nod silently, and place the tubes back down beside her chair. As *Texas Justice* proceeds on the television, I consider how little I know about Dorothy's medical condition. I've been visiting her for 4 months, and most of the time she seems to be getting better, not worse. Then, out of the blue, she has trouble with an activity she has performed automatically hundreds of times. I don't even know if Dorothy's confusion is something I need to worry about.

When I turn to look at her, Dorothy smiles and shakes her head.

"I wonder if these people know just how stupid they look when they come on television like this," she says.

"You're right, Dorothy," I reply. "They're pretty crazy."

"They're crazy all right," Dorothy says.

After a moment, she asks, "How are those kids at the school behaving? Not giving you any trouble, I hope."

"They keep me busy, that's for sure," I reply, smiling. "They're generally very good."

"That's good to hear," Dorothy says, completing our ritualized exchange about my teaching. "Would you like some of that coffee now?" she asks.

"Sure," I reply, "I'll get it."

"You know where to find everything," she says. "Just make yourself at home."

As I pour our coffee, I do feel at home in Dorothy's apartment, and I do feel comfortable with her. And yet, I also feel uncomfortable with her illness and I wonder why it seems "against the rules" for me to talk about it with her.

BUILDING A BRIDGE

Dorothy and I are sitting in the Crossroads Diner; we rarely go anywhere else to eat anymore. She is eating her usual ham and cheese omelet and I have my fish sandwich and fries.

"I know something I wanted to tell you," Dorothy says, suddenly.

"What's that, Dorothy?" I ask.

"You know Terry's daughter, Leslie?" she asks.

"Yes," I reply. "I've met her a couple of times when she stayed at your apartment."

"Did I tell you about that no-good husband of hers?" Dorothy asks.

"You told me a little," I reply.

"Well, Leslie kicked him out of the house," Dorothy announces. "They're getting a divorce."

I can't tell how she feels about this, but I sense she wants to talk about it, so I ask, "How do you feel about that, Dorothy?"

"He wasn't a very good husband," she begins. "When people got married in my day, it was for life, none of this shacking up together and having babies and so on. But the thing is, Leslie has a right to be happy. I don't think she should have married that no good son-of-a-bitch in the first place—if you'll pardon my language. So, maybe it's the right thing that they're splitting up."

I nod quietly. I think about the fact that I am divorced. I wonder what Dorothy would think about my situation. I'm comforted that she seems to accept what's happening with Leslie, and I decide to tell her about me.

"I used to be married, too, Dorothy," I say. "Not for very long, but we got divorced."

Dorothy looks at me for a moment and then says gently, "I didn't know that."

"I don't really mention it, because sometimes I feel embarrassed about it," I say. I feel myself wanting her to understand, although I'm not sure why I brought it up. "When I got married, I thought it would be for life, like you and Stan. But the man I married didn't feel the same way about it."

"That's not your fault," Dorothy says, firmly. "It takes two to make a marriage like mine and Stan's, and I'm not even saying that our marriage was the best. We had some really hard times. But if your husband didn't want to be a husband, then you're better off without him."

"Thank you for saying that, Dorothy," I appreciate her sincere efforts to comfort and accept me, despite her upbringing and her apparent misgivings about divorce.

We eat in silence for a minute or two, and then Dorothy says, "You know Terry's other daughter, Sharon? She and Leslie have different fathers. Terry was married before, too."

"She's never mentioned that," I reply.

"Well, she wouldn't," Dorothy says. "It was a long time ago, but there it is. You see? It can happen to anybody."

Dorothy continues to eat her omelet, and I am happy for that to be the last word on the subject. I feel as if, suddenly, a bridge has appeared between us. We may have been building this bridge for months, but it only became visible once we stepped forward and realized that it is strong enough to hold us.

After lunch, Dorothy and I return to her apartment and hang out in the breezeway for a little while. When it is time for me to go, she stands up from her chair and we hug for the first time.

"Thanks for a wonderful lunch, Dorothy," I say as we embrace.

Dorothy's hands rest lightly on my shoulders and she replies, "I enjoyed it! I always enjoy our visits, I hope you know that."

"I'm glad," I reply. "I always enjoy them, too.

"You be careful now," Dorothy says as I start to walk to my car. "There are a lot of crazy drivers out there."

"I promise I'll be careful," I reply and wave. I smile all the way home.

TOM

Since our first interview, Tom has moved to his new house on Tampa Bay, a few miles from where he had lived previously. As I drive into the subdivision, I notice that many of the homes are still under construction, but Tom's place is finished. After a brief tour, during which we discuss the relative merits of different floorings and faux finish paint textures, Tom and I settle into his comfortable living room, and begin. I remind Tom about the magazine pictures of flowers he cut out and put on his patient's notice board.

Tom explains, "She went downhill quickly after that. After that visit, I went once and I didn't stay very long. Then, Patrice called me and said she took a turn for the worse. I went to see her and the only thing she really said was, 'I don't know what's happening. I don't know what's going on.' I thought after seeing her, and what Patrice said, that there wasn't a lot of time left. I guess it was 2 to 3 weeks after the last interview that she passed away."

"How did you respond to that, both emotionally and practically?"

"Well, it was kind of a shock. My patient was really bad at first, then she seemed to be getting better every time I went so I felt good. I knew that it probably didn't have anything to do with me, but maybe she was adjusting to the nursing home. Then, when she took a turn for the worse, I felt kind of lost. She was in so much pain. How she was living at the end, it didn't seem like she had any kind of life at all. I know she had children who did not come to see her. I always wondered about that. It was sad, but it didn't seem like a bad thing that she passed away. I knew she was really sick, but I couldn't tell that she was dying. In my own mind, I thought she might just be having a bad day."

I feel sad for Tom, because I know how hard he tried to help his patient, and then he was caught off guard by her death. I comment, "It is really hard to know, I suppose. How do you know when it's going to be the last time you see somebody?"

Tom replies, "I think I expected her to be on a ventilator, or have tubes coming out of her and nurses trying to keep her alive for a couple of weeks before she died, but that never happened. I guess I'm thinking of television and movies where they have lights and monitors and stuff like that, so maybe it made me think it wasn't time yet."

"How do you feel about the last visit and the role you played in her life?"

"I didn't think I made that big a difference, when I look back on it," Tom says, shrugging a little. "I remember her being really happy and she talked to me when I brought the flowers and put them up for her. Then I knew that I'd done something good for her. Overall, I don't know how much I helped."

I comment, "It sounds like she was in more pain than she should have been, ideally, from a hospice perspective. Her pain seems to have been the main obstacle to having a relationship with her, because she didn't have the energy to engage with you."

Tom nods, "That makes sense. That's why I was so medical about my notes. I just knew that she needed help with her pain. Whereas now, apparently my patient doesn't have a pain problem, so I don't mention it."

"So, you took a short break after your first patient, then got a call from Patrice?"

"Yes. Patrice had two patients and she asked me to pick one."

From our telephone conversation, I already know what Tom's choice was. I smile. "So, why did you pick the 99-year-old fellow in the nursing home?"

Tom smiles back at me. "Because she told me he didn't have any family. I knew the other gentleman had a family and would get a volunteer, maybe not right away, but eventually. The other person seemed to have a much greater need."

I nod. "Now, this was the patient you told me you've been seeing for a while but they haven't got a clear diagnosis for him?"

"Right. It's been 4 months and I haven't seen a nurse, chaplain, social worker."

"You go, you write your notes—" I prompt.

"I go, I write my notes, I make my copy, I put it in the mail, and then it's the weekend again. I feel like I'm freelancing—like hospice forgot about me," Tom laughs. "He's not in pain, but I'm concerned that he thinks his legs will get better and he'll go back to where he was before. He is very 'with it.' He makes more sense than half the people I work with. He'll tell me about land deals he made in 1920, about the Titanic, people he met. He is the total opposite of the last patient I had. I'll walk in and he's all smiles. He'll start talking and 3 hours later he'll stop."

"Wow. You go to visit him for that long?"

"Yeah. I mostly stay 3½ hours, usually on the weekend. The nursing home smells *really* bad, but Patrice said you can't judge it by that. The first one had chandeliers and a beautiful restaurant, but I never saw a nurse go in and check on my patient. This one is very basic. He has a bed, a drawer. The last one had a television in every room. He has nothing. It's an indigent nursing home; there are a lot of people there who used to live on the street. But after saying all that, someone will go in every 10 minutes—a nurse or a doctor—bringing him juice or water. If you need anything, they're there right away. The care is awesome. In the palace over there, they don't care. The staff are all out in the hall talking or laughing."

"For profit versus not for profit," I comment.

"Exactly," Tom agrees. "I think he first went to an ALF [assisted living facility] and they didn't expect him to live for so long. His body works from the neck up. From the neck down, he can move his arms and hands a little bit, but he can't stand up. I think all his money went to the ALF and they couldn't handle him any more, then the nursing home took him in."

"So, Patrice told you about this fellow in the nursing home and prepared you for what that would be like. Why don't you tell me about the first visit?"

Tom begins: "I pulled up in the parking lot and had to decide whether I should even go in. There were people all over the parking lot in wheelchairs, smoking, and wheeling themselves around. I walked in, and right away it smelled really bad. And people were crying and making sounds like cats and dogs. It was more like you would think of an asylum than a nursing home. So, I found him and explained I was from hospice. I said, 'Nurse Donna thought you might like me to come and see you.' I ended up being there for about half an hour, partly because the whole situation was kind of a shock to me. The next time I went to see him, I explained who I was again. I stayed for about 2 hours. He talked to me but it was fairly awkward. The third time, he remembered who I was, but not really. He said, 'Oh, you again. You're not the doctor, are you?' By the fourth time I walked in, he knew exactly who I was," Tom smiles.

Tom leans forward as if he's leaning in toward his patient. "All he has on him is this little, thin blanket, it can't weigh more than a pound, but the blanket is so heavy to him that he can't roll over by himself. So, when I go visit I'll lift up the blanket and he'll roll over so he can get into a comfortable position to see me. Then, nonstop, he'll talk, talk, talk."

"Do you bring the chair next to the bed?" I ask.

Tom nods. "I pull the chair up to the bed and we'll just talk. We never talk about his medical condition, and that's why I'm kind of concerned. Obviously the hospice nurses come because I ask and he'll say, 'Oh, yes, Donna came today.' From what I can figure out, his doctor put him on the program because he was in a nursing home, and he's lonely, and he's old. The only thing terminal about him is that he's 99."

"You mean they declared him to be terminal because of probability?"

"Right. And he eats whatever he likes; he has cookies; he has his vitamins chopped up in apple sauce; he has milk; he likes milkshakes. He has a real nice wheelchair that sits there in the corner, and he just knows he's going to get back in that wheelchair as soon as he gets the strength back in his legs—but that's not going to happen."

"How do you respond to that?"

Tom shrugs. "I just listen to him and say, 'Well, you keep doing your exercises there in the bed.' He fell, and they took his walker away from him. He says, 'I knew if I stayed in that wheelchair too long, I'd never get out of it. Now, it's going to be even harder for me, because I have to get back in the wheelchair first and then into the walker.' And he keeps thinking he's going to go back to the ALF because he liked it better there. I told him that the other place I was at, the staff didn't take care of anybody. I said, 'You can see that these people really care; they're in here all the time. In the other place, I never saw anybody even stick their head in the door.'"

I smile. "What did he say?"

"He liked it," Tom says with a grin and nods. "He smiled and said, 'So I picked the right place, huh?' He has a great personality. I just keep thinking that the average stay in hospice is 2 months—well, I think after that, they start looking at whether this person is right for hospice. That's my biggest fear because there is no way I will stop seeing him as often as I am now. I don't really have time to see two patients, so I'll just tell hospice I'm ready for another patient and I'll see both, although I'll just be seeing one officially."

"Why do you think it's important for you to keep going?" I prompt.

"I think he enjoys me visiting him. He lives in this room all by himself without television, without newspaper, without magazines, no contact other than the people who come to give him food and give him a bath. I can't imagine leaving him without anybody."

"I don't know what to make of that," I ponder. "On the one hand, I think the hospice people who first assessed him may not realize how healthy he is. But on the other hand, he still needs the company even though he may not be an 'appropriate' hospice patient."

"He needs a volunteer from *somewhere*," Tom agrees.

"Well, that leads me to a question about your relationship with him. Do you think of him, like you said, as a friend? Or do you think of him more as a family member?"

"You know," Tom responds thoughtfully. "I think of him as a family member, mainly because of my uncle. My uncle was put in a nursing home about 5 years ago and I never went to see him. He was there for 5 months and he died there. Maybe when I go to see my patient now, I see what my uncle saw, and I think, 'This could have been my uncle sitting here with nothing, looking at these four walls.' I feel now like I'm visiting my uncle, and I'm making up for a time when I should have visited my relative and I didn't."

Tom's story makes me think about my great aunt. The same year that my grandmother died, my great aunt died in a nursing home after a series of strokes. I confess to Tom that as my aunt's physical and mental deterioration progressed, I only ever visited her with my younger brother, Andy.

Unlike me, Andy seemed to know exactly what to say and do. He knew how to just be there with Auntie Poppy. Sporting spiky orange or purple hair, he chatted about the rave parties and nightclubs he played with his band. He wheeled Poppy out to the garden and brushed her soft white hair. I didn't know how to initiate those things with her, and I felt incapable of the relaxed tenderness that came so easily for Andy. I waited too long between visits, and I didn't get to say goodbye before she passed away. I feel ashamed of the way I neglected my great aunt once she went into the nursing home. I consider myself to be empathic and caring, but I couldn't see past my own discomfort and sadness in order to respond compassionately to my aunt. I'm convinced that I would respond to her differently now than I did back then. It's validating to know that Tom has had a similar experience and found himself changed.

Tom continues: "I feel protective of him. He told me once that they didn't give him a toothbrush, and I said, 'Why? Aren't you allowed to have one?' And he said, 'Yes, I'm allowed to have one.' I was mad. I asked the nurse, 'Why doesn't he have a toothbrush?' And she said, 'We give him one almost every other day, but he keeps losing them. We have no idea what he does with them.'"

I start laughing because it sounds so ridiculous. "But he doesn't go anywhere!"

Tom starts chuckling, too. "Yeah! So I'm trying to look behind the bed to see if I can find a pile of toothbrushes. I felt a bit guilty because I'd jumped on the nurse a little bit and she'd been doing her job all along. I wrote it on one of the notes for hospice, 'I'm concerned he's not getting a toothbrush, but the nurse says he keeps losing them. We may want to follow up on that.' That's the closest I've come to a medical type of note."

"So, does he know what hospice is? That hospice is for people who are dying?"

"Yes," Tom replies with a playful expression that suggests there is more to tell.

"How do you know that?" I probe.

"Because he said, 'You know they think I'm terminal. What do you think?'"

"Oh my God!" I exclaim in disbelief.

Tom grins. "And I said, 'I guess you are. And so am I. From the time we take our first breath we're terminal. We're going to die eventually.' And he said, 'Yep, that's true.' That's how I got by that one," Tom smiles and rolls his eyes. "Another time he said that the priest came by. He said, 'He gave me my last rites. Do you think they're trying to tell me something?'"

I start laughing again. I can't help myself. "So he's joking about it?"

"Yeah!" Tom replies. "I said, 'Are you sure he didn't come to give you communion or confession?' He said, 'I think that was my last rites. I think they're trying to tell me something.'"

"Well, it seems he's not depressed. Would that be accurate?" I ask. "He's lonely, and he's a little frustrated that he's in bed, but not depressed."

"No," Tom replies, more seriously. "But before I go into the room, I always look to see if he's sleeping. The first day, he asked me not to wake him if he's sleeping because the staff always wakes him up. So, maybe twice I went by and he was asleep, and I said, 'Yeah, I came by the other day and you were sleeping.' The second time that happened, he said, 'Let's forget that. If you come by, just wake me up.' Today he was very soundly asleep so I didn't wake him."

"Will you tell him you were there or ...."

"No, I won't tell him," Tom says, smiling gently. "Sometimes when I go and I look in, he'll look very depressed, very sad. When I walk in, he gets this big smile on his face and says, 'There you are! How are you? Crank the bed up! Crank the bed up! Let me get a better look at you.'"

"What's been the best thing about volunteering?"

"I'd say meeting this patient and knowing that, with this guy, I've made a difference. I leave there thinking I really helped him, and it makes me happy. I don't want to say that it's a spiritual thing, but in my mind, it gets into that."

"Well, here's a question for you, Tom," I say, leaning forward. "You're talking about these visits as something he looks forward to and as something that's potentially keeping him alive. But, isn't it our job to help the end transition to be easier?"

Tom smiles and shifts a little uncomfortably in his seat. "It is," he speaks slowly and deliberately. "But I think in my situation with my patient, my *unique* patient, who is *not* going through that .... It was very clear with the other lady, I was trying to make sure she was comfortable and that she had some joy in her life. But I knew she was dying. When you asked that question, I thought, 'He's not going to die. I'm going to be seeing him until I'm 50.'"

"Yeah," I say, unconvinced. "What if his condition changes and he becomes very ill?"

"I think the whole relationship would change," Tom replies. "Because right now the relationship is all about being friends; then the relationship would revolve more around his last days and making sure he was as comfortable as possible."

I wonder: "Do you feel that all the discussions you have are establishing the kind of relationship where you could talk about dying with him?"

"I have no doubt that he totally trusts me. When I first went there, he wouldn't say too much. But now he'll tell me things; he trusts me to be the bad guy with little things like the toothbrush and other things that bothered him that I took care of. I think he knows that I'm not going anywhere, too. He knows I'll always be there to stick up for him. I don't know how I know that, but I get that feeling.

"Before I started, I was expecting to be dealing more with people dying. And it's so totally not that. I was expecting it to be more spiritual than it is. But I'm not disappointed; I don't want to sway our conversations that way."

I respond: "I'd always framed this work as something that I couldn't do because it was emotionally overwhelming. It's a big surprise to me how human and ordinary this work is—what we do and the things that we talk about. It's about living, and trying to respond to that life in the best way possible. It sounds as though that's just what being with him is like."

Tom and I sit in silence for a few moments and then I say, "I hope you get to quietly continue seeing your hospice patient. Is there anything we haven't covered?"

"Not really, nothing I can think of," Tom says smiling.

We talk briefly about the possibility of another interview, then Tom walks me out to my car and I drive home along the bay as the sky darkens into night. I think about how committed Tom is to his patient and his assertion that he will continue to visit him even if he is taken off the hospice program. Dorothy's condition seems to have stabilized and although her diagnosis is specific—unlike Tom's patient's—her prognosis is not. Could Dorothy graduate from hospice a second time? I feel uneasy about the idea that there is an appropriate hospice patient. Even if hospice decides that Tom's patient and Dorothy no longer qualify as dying, they may still need us to visit with them. Even if Dorothy is dying, we never talk about it, so the dying process as defined by hospice obviously doesn't impact my relationship with Dorothy all that much.

I examine my logic and recognize that Tom and I define our relationships with our patients as more or less distinct from hospice. Hospice brought us together, but as time has passed we define our role in terms of who we are to each other, not in terms of what is appropriate for hospice. Of course, the hospice approach also allows flexibility and individual interpretation within the roles of the team. Perhaps that means that it is okay for Tom and me to forget that our patients are dying, and to define our relationships with our patients as distinct from the idea of end of life care. In any case, if our patients do graduate, I sense that Tom and I feel right about following our hearts first and the rules second.

SARAH

I meet Sarah in her office in the Aging Studies Department at the University of South Florida for our second interview. As we settle into our chairs, I am aware of how small and quiet the room is, with no windows and few distractions. The environment urges me to get down to business. I remind Sara that in our last conversation, she said her patient "could go on and on."

Sarah shrugs and shakes her head a little as she begins. "She hasn't lost weight, eats normally, goes out. She has grandkids and great-grandkids who visit; they are remodeling the house. She's very active! I think she's going to live 4 or 5 years, I really do."

Dorothy's condition has remained essentially unchanged for the past few months. I begin to compare Sarah's interpretation of her patient's health with my own thoughts about Dorothy.

I ask: "Does your patient acknowledge her illness? Or do you think that because she's not too sick she doesn't have to think about it?"

"I think because she's not so sick she doesn't have to think about it," Sarah replies confidently. "She didn't go to her family reunion because of her health. It's something they do every year, but I think that's the only sign that things are different for her now. Other than that, her daughter lives with her, they have dinner at night, they watch TV together, they go out. Being a hospice patient doesn't necessarily mean the same to her as someone who's lying in a nursing home bed, barely breathing. She's also been told by the hospice nurse—it's the same thing I told her when she asked me—that she's going to live for a couple of years."

"That's what you told her?" I ask because Dorothy and I have never talked about it in this way, and I'm surprised that Sarah could be that direct about her patient's condition.

"Yeah."

"So she asked you explicitly?"

"She asked me explicitly what I thought and I said, 'Honestly, congestive heart failure, 50% is not bad.' No one had told her up to that point what that really means. Apparently, she asked the hospice nurse, and then she asked me. It's something I study, so I happened to know what congestive heart failure is, what the success rates are, and I know that there's nothing they can do about it, so I gave her the information. 'Congestive heart failure is degenerative. Right now, for you to become bedridden, it's generally a 4- or 5-year process, as long as you take care of yourself. But you could have a heart attack tomorrow and die, if you're not careful.' I explained to her that the more stress you put on your heart, the faster you're going to die, it's just that simple. It's strange that no one explained that to her."

Because Sarah's patient appears to be relatively healthy, another thought occurs to me. I observe: "We've been with our patients for about 5 months and I've started to be concerned because my patient hasn't shown too many signs of deterioration recently. I began to worry that they might suspend her from the program."

Sarah picks up on my thought immediately. "I've thought about that, too. What's good and what's bad in the work that I do is that I know exactly how LifePath functions. I know the business side behind the personal side. My patient has to be rediagnosed after 6 months, and she's definitely not worse than she was 6 months ago. She's not *better*, but I don't think she's worse. If she gets taken off the program, it would be very sad."

"What would you do?"

Now I'm thinking about Tom's response to the same concern. He was emphatic that he would continue to visit his patient no matter what hospice said or did.

Sarah responds thoughtfully. "I probably wouldn't see her weekly, because I don't think that's appropriate. But I would definitely keep her phone number, and give her a call every couple of weeks just to say hi, and see how she's doing. She might want to see me, but I probably wouldn't do that out of respect for hospice and wanting to remain a volunteer for the organization. But I would definitely stay in touch, and I'd stop by to see her once a month, but not once a week."

I share Tom's story with Sarah and it occurs to me that the social networks of the two patients are very different, which might affect how each feels about his or her relationship. I conclude Tom's story with an observation. "I may be wrong, but my impression is that because your patient has an active system of family support, it might be easier for you to leave. Maybe it's been easier for you to maintain boundaries with your patient now. Would that be correct?"

"Absolutely. If you're the only person the patient sees, then of course that's a totally different thing. With someone who has visitors and family who live in the area, you're not abandoning them to be by themselves. In Tom's situation, I would have a really hard time not seeing a person regularly after they leave hospice."

"One of the things I talked about with Tom is the reward we get from doing this. I thought that in Tom's relationship with his patient, he might start feeling burdened. But he said that he doesn't, partly because this guy is so glad to see him when he comes, and also the give and take of the friendship that they've established. What about with your patient?"

"For me, it's definitely reciprocal," Sarah agrees. "I can honestly say that if it's been 2 weeks since we've seen each other, when I walk through the door, she's happy that I'm there and I'm happy to be there. Despite the rules about not sharing any of your own information, I can't do that. My patient shares her life with me, and out of respect for that, I tell her things about my family. I think I get a whole lot out of it."

I reflect, "Emilia visited a patient with Alzheimer's and she spent the whole time wheeling her patient around the nursing home. Emilia said that, as active as it was, it was almost like meditation—she left feeling more grounded and grateful for her life."

Sarah pauses for a moment, thinking. "My patient is very different from me. It makes me very grateful for my own family and also very thankful for all the people in my life who care about me and listen to me. Definitely, when I go there, everything else disappears. Sometimes there's something that I just can't let go of, but for the most part, when I'm there I think about my patient—that she's comfortable with me and that everything is fine."

Again, Sarah's observations echo my experiences of visiting Dorothy.

Sarah continues, "Visiting my patient also helps me to realize how young I really am and how much life I have ahead of me. How many chances do you get to meet someone who is nearly 60 years older than you are, who reflects on her life with you? I definitely feel that I'm grounded—that's a really good way of putting it—I feel very grounded when I leave there."

Sarah's response also makes me think about the ways that our patients have become integrated into our lives, and yet are not really a part of them. I tell Sarah, "When I visit Dorothy, I find it easier to leave other stuff at the door than I do leaving her behind when I leave. It sounds like you don't totally leave your patient at the door either, because you said that when you haven't seen her for a couple of weeks, you look forward to coming back. But we're supposed to be preparing ourselves for our patients' deaths, not developing feelings that will make it harder for us to let go. How do we find balance between caring and maintaining distance?"

Sarah shakes her head slightly, confirming my hunch that she has thought about this, too. "Part of it for me is that the thought that she could die doesn't even register. If there were to be signs of rapid deterioration, then yes, but it's hard to see her as someone who's all that sick. I definitely don't leave her there and not think about her at all, but she also doesn't stay on my mind all the time. I'll call her and have a conversation; I look forward to spending time with her, but I don't want to be that integrated into her life because I don't think that's fair. I should be a visitor, a friend, a volunteer, but not another granddaughter. I think if I felt like each visit might be the last time I see her, it would be different. But I don't, and that makes it easier, because I always assume that the next week I'm going to talk to her again."

"Are you prepared for her worst case scenario?" I ask.

"I don't think I'm prepared for a worst case scenario, because I don't think you really can be. Even from my personal experience with my grandfather, you can have years of knowing that this is going to happen, and when it comes, it's a complete other feeling. You can be logical and you can be reasonable and rational, but you can't predict your emotions—I can't anyway."

"So, how do you feel about your relationship?" I prompt.

"She likes to share her experiences and her past with me. She talks a lot about herself and her husband when the kids were young. The family has heard it a thousand times, or they've lived through it, so it's not really conversation that she has with them."

I wonder if Sarah, as an aging studies scholar, has considered the functions of life review in end-of-life communication. "Do you have any sense of what that means to her, particularly as a hospice patient?"

Sarah nods. "It's important because when you get to be a certain age, you think about your past and your life as a whole, but you don't get to share it very much. She also realizes that although she may be getting sick now, she's had a good life: a lot of family, a lot of friends, a great husband, great experiences, a great job. So, a lot of it is acceptance and going back over the great things in her life and reliving them. She's not going to go out again and get another job. She'll never again be at the point where she doesn't need the wheelchair when she goes to the grocery store. I think having someone listen to her stories makes her not feel as badly that she's at this stage where her life is coming to a close."

"So, would you say that's an important part of communicating with people who are dying?" I ask, trying to identify distinctions among aging, end-of-life, and dying.

Sarah clarifies her position. "Again, I don't think she fits the definition of someone who is dying, but a lot of our conversations are about the past. A lot of my communication involves listening and communicating parts of myself without going overboard. I think there's a trick to it. If you can share your experiences so that it's reciprocal, and the patient feels it's a give and take, and it's not just you sitting there on the couch like a shrink. Learning how to give part of yourself, because they are giving part of themselves to you, is really important."

I recall my conversation with Dorothy where I told her I was divorced; it was a true moment of connection between us.

Sarah continues, "When I talk to my patient, I always make sure that I look her in the eye. I make sure when we're speaking that I'm not looking off somewhere else, so she knows she has my attention. No matter what the condition of our patients, they need to know that you're *really there*. Even if they can't talk and they're not communicative, if a patient is there lying in bed and you're just there just to keep her company, you let her know that."

Again, I think of Dorothy—of us sitting together in the breezeway, in silence, together.

Sarah leans forward a little in her chair and explains, "From the very beginning, I think what made it easy for her to trust me was that she saw I wasn't asking her the same questions. I remembered family members' names; I wasn't going through the motions with her. So, I think the two big secrets are learning to share yourself so that you're not just an ear, you're a partner in the relationship, and then let them trust you so they can talk about whatever they want to talk about. They're both very important."

I think out loud. "You mentioned reciprocity earlier on and that is something that surprised me. I originally thought of volunteering as giving to the patient. But receiving the gifts that she has to offer has meant so much to me. Dorothy has these little wisdoms, things about life that she shares with me. I don't care if I hear them a hundred times. I love to listen to her. It's nice to feel like I'm bringing something to her life, but *she* gives a lot to *me*."

Sarah adds to my thought, "And it's also consistency. I'm consistently there. She knows that every Thursday I'll be there, and if I can't do it Thursday, I do it Wednesday or Friday. I've developed a pattern; I call her the morning that I'm going to see her. I never let her down. I tell her if I'm going to be out of town. I don't just skip it; I try to reschedule so she doesn't feel like she's lost touch. And I think that's also really important."

As we approach the end of the interview, I ask, "Has there been a real bright spark or a positive aspect of your volunteering so far that stands out to you?"

Sarah responds, "For me, it's not often that I come across someone who has a need in their life that I can actually fulfill. It makes me feel good to be able to give that to someone. To find a part of your week, a part of your life, that is available for them, and that's the best part—absolutely. I may run across 50 people in the day and have random conversations, but it's not the same as this interaction. It's important to her and it's important to me. That's the best thing."

I think about my relationship with Dorothy and I agree with Sarah. On one level, I could say that Dorothy and I simply hang out together and go out to lunch—very ordinary and mundane types of activities—and it would not express the significance of the moments that we share. It seems so easy now that sometimes I forget how important these hours are for Dorothy, and for me.

As I consider the tone and topics of these interviews with Tom and Sarah, as compared to the first interviews 6 months ago, I am fascinated by how our attitudes about volunteering have changed. Of course, it comes as no surprise that our relationships with our patients have changed over time as unique relational cultures have emerged through our interaction. What does surprise me is how different these stories are from what we had anticipated at the beginning. Sarah, who expressed some initial misgivings about the personal nature of hospice volunteering at the beginning of the year, in this interview advocated reciprocity as a means of developing a trusting and worthwhile relationship. Tom, who was initially drawn to hospice because he was interested in death and providing comfort to people who were dying, is now enjoying a friendship with a patient who appears to be disabled but not necessarily dying. I also note with interest that despite his initial motivation for volunteering, Tom did not engage in a conversation about death when his patient brought up the subject of being terminal. As for me, I realize that I have fallen into the routine of going out to lunch with Dorothy, although that was the last thing I envisioned doing as a volunteer.

Although our activities with our patients have evolved in response to their unique personalities, needs, and physical capabilities, I can also see that we have not left behind the hospice framework for our relationships. Clearly, all three of us are happy to be involved with our patients and feel that there is value in what we are doing, and yet there seems to be an undercurrent of doubt that we are authentic volunteers, because our patients do not conform to our concepts of people who are dying. Even as we strive to be in the present moment with our patients, it seems that upon reflection we each think about the ending of the relationship—not to death, as we expected, but to the graduation of our patients from the hospice program. I feel an inherent contradiction between the natural emergence and development of our relationships with our patients and the overarching supervision of these relationships by hospice as an organization. Perhaps because Sarah is more knowledgeable about the clinical aspects of end-of-life care, she has spoken explicitly with her patient about her condition—but Tom and I have not. Instead, Tom and I perform "as if" hospice was not an element of our relationships with our patients. Despite our concerns about our patients being taken off the program, we act "as if" these relationships will not end at all. I find it hard to decide whether Tom and I are merely following the rules of improvisation and staying in the moment, or if we are ignoring the reality of hospice because it is easier for us to do so.

"THE" CONVERSATION

Dorothy has been doing well ever since what Jackie, Dorothy's nurse, described as her "spell" with the coffee pot 2 months ago. I never see her using her oxygen, although she tells me she still uses it at night, when she sleeps. Len has another week off, and when I arrive at the apartment, I learn that he took Terry and Dorothy out to a comedy club over the weekend. Dorothy is thoroughly delighted as she tells me about the acts she saw and the other people they met up with at the show. At first, I worry about the smoke in the comedy club, but then I see how happy Dorothy is to have had some excitement brought into her life with a rare night out. I tell Len that I think the club was a wonderful idea.

"We had a good old time, didn't we, Dorothy?" Len says.

"We sure did," Dorothy grins.

It is raining today, and Dorothy says she would like to watch the rain, so we all go out to sit in the breezeway. Other than the Crossroads Diner, I believe this must be Dorothy's favorite place to spend time.

After a few minutes more of talking about the comedy club, Len says, "Terry, wasn't there something you wanted to ask this young lady about hospice?"

Len is still unsure about how to pronounce my name, so he doesn't use it at all.

"Right," Terry replies. "I wanted to ask if you have any other numbers for hospice."

"You mean, other than the office numbers?" I ask.

"I mean for an emergency," Terry clarifies.

"I have the numbers for my volunteer coordinator," I say, "but that's not what you would use in an emergency. Are you worried about something?"

"Nothing bad has happened yet," Terry explains, "but every time I need something from hospice, like medicine, or if Mom's nurse doesn't show up one day, I use the main office number. Well, I tell them what the problem is and they say someone will call me back. Half the time I don't get a call back until the next day or the day after that, and sometimes they *never* call! So, it occurred to me that if something were to happen to Mom, it would be useless to use that office number, because nobody would call back. Do you know what I'm saying? They said that I'm supposed to call hospice first, but I've decided that I'm going to call 9-1-1, because I just don't think hospice will respond the way they should."

A hundred thoughts are running through my head at once and a hundred problems that I'm not sure how to address. I decide to ask for clarification.

"What kind of emergency are you thinking about where you would need 9-1-1?" I ask.

"They gave me this kit when Mom first went into hospice," Terry explains. "It's an emergency kit in case she has an attack, but I'm not even sure how to use it. I think that's why I'm supposed to call hospice. But, like I said, I'm going to call 9-1-1, because at least I know that they will come to help me."

It sounds to me like Terry is talking about a respiratory attack of some kind or sudden heart failure. My mind goes to the yellow DNR (Do Not Resuscitate) order stuck on the refrigerator with little plastic fruit magnets. Although hospice does not require that patients sign a DNR order to be admitted to hospice, it can help to clarify the nature of hospice care for the patients and family, as well as to notify outside medical professionals—such as emergency technicians and hospital staff—about the wishes of a hospice patient. Dorothy signed the DNR order when she joined the hospice program, and it notifies the 9-1-1 team and the doctors at the hospital *not* to administer any lifesaving measures. So, now I am confused about what Terry expects to happen in the case of Dorothy having "an attack." Jackie, Dorothy's hospice nurse, has alluded to Dorothy being "in denial." Now I'm worried that Terry and Dorothy don't understand what hospice is for.

"I understand that you feel frustrated about hospice not returning your calls," I say. "I'll definitely call to complain about that because you shouldn't be left hanging, but I'm also worried about you calling 9-1-1. You have a signed DNR order on your refrigerator; do you understand what that means in terms of calling 9-1-1 and going to the hospital?"

I feel very hesitant and nervous. I've never talked about Dorothy's illness in this way before, and certainly never talked about anything to do with her death.

After sitting silently in her chair since we came outside, Dorothy suddenly pipes up. "I know what that means," she replies. "It means that they won't put me on any machines, and that's fine with me. When The Man Upstairs calls your number, it's your time and there's nothing you can do about it, so I don't want to be stuck in the hospital on some machine."

I breathe a silent sigh of relief. "Okay, then, Dorothy," I respond. "I just wanted to make sure that was okay with you."

"Right," Terry says, "it means they'll make her comfortable but they won't do anything to prolong her life."

"That's exactly right," I say. I feel myself relax a little.

Terry continues, "But what I'm worried about is getting into a situation with Mom where I need help. I don't want to be here all alone waiting for hours for someone to return my call."

"And you shouldn't have to," I say, emphatically. "Would you let me call hospice about that? The best thing would be to get a hospice nurse out to you quickly so you don't have to go to the hospital, but you should feel free to call 9-1-1 if you don't have the support that you need."

I want to defend hospice and argue that a hospitalization would be the worst thing to happen for Dorothy. Even with a signed DNR order, if an emergency team and hospital staff are unfamiliar with Dorothy's case and circumstances, it is very likely that Dorothy would be put onto a respirator until the hospital could discuss her status with Terry and other family members. I don't want Dorothy's care to be put into the hands of strangers in a hospital, and I don't want Terry to have to face the decision of taking Dorothy off life support, so part of me wants to argue against their plan. At the same time, I feel very protective of Terry and Dorothy. I'm upset because the hospice communication system has failed to meet their needs, and I also feel helpless because I don't know enough about how the system works. I can't even reassure them that there is a procedure in which emergency cases get handled immediately and nonurgent questions—like the ones they've had so far—have to wait. I vow to find out as soon as I get home.

"I'd appreciate you making that call," Terry responds.

"I promise I will," I say.

"Looks like it's clearing up," Dorothy says, still looking out at the sky. "Do you feel like a bite to eat? Maybe we could all go down to the Crossroads Diner."

It appears that Dorothy is still in party mode. "Sure," I reply. "That'd be great."

REFLECTIONS: WHAT DOES IT MEAN TO BE "DYING" IN HOSPICE?

In this reflection, I focus on one aspect of the volunteer role that re- quired us to improvise while coming to terms with an unanticipated source of uncertainty in hospice; specifically, the question of when someone is dying. In chapter 1, I observed that the word *hospice* con- notes multiple meanings and may be seen as operating at three distinct levels. First, hospice is a social movement and a philosophy of end-of-life care. Second, it is a *type* of organization as well as a *specific* or- ganization such as LifePath Hospice and Palliative Care. Third, it is a subjective construction of an individual volunteer, hospice worker, pa- tient, or family member. At various times throughout the interviews, the volunteers referred to each of these meanings of hospice, and often these different layers of hospice merged and affected our experiences of volunteering. Sometimes conflicts arose when two or more of these lay- ers contradicted each other; for example, when our responses to a pa- tient conformed to our understanding of hospice-as-philosophy, but contradicted the guidelines of the organization— as in Tom's special case of visiting his patient who was (according to Tom) "not dying." Conversely, as in my situation with Dorothy and the 9-1-1 call, conflict arose when I found myself called upon to act as a hospice representative while not fully understanding the organization or the specific cases that Terry described when her calls were not returned. In reflecting on the significance of the stories in this chapter, it is necessary for me to speak to the different "layers" of hospice (as philosophy, as organization, and as experienced by the volunteers) because, as we learned, the determi- nation of whether someone is dying is as much a symbolic construction of the organization as it is an empirically determined state. When it is necessary to distinguish one of these connotations of hospice from the other two, I will identify the particular usage I intend by applying one of the following terms: hospice-as-philosophy, hospice-as-organization, or hospice-as-experienced.

As illustrated by the stories in this chapter, at several points throughout this research, the other volunteers and I encountered dying as it related to the intersection of hospice services and our relationships with our patients. Some volunteers had patients who died within days of the first visit, and other patients lived for several months. As she predicted in her interview, Sarah's patient eventually graduated from hospice; her services were reduced and then suspended, until some time in the future when she might become eligible again. All hospice patients are by definition dying, but the diversity of our experiences attests to the fact that *dying* is a socially constructed (Berger & Luckmann, 1967) category, and is far more ambiguous than our common usage of the word suggests. Indeed, researchers in aging and end-of-life studies now recognize dying as a social process as well as a physical event (Bradley, Fried, Kasl, & Idler, 2000; Lawton, 2000; Seale, 1998). This is an important shift in our cultural understanding of death and dying, which I will address more fully at the end of Part IV. First, though, I want to focus on the aspects of the stories in this chapter that demonstrate how the concept of dying tended to revolve around two very practical concerns—dying as an impending physical reality that affected interpersonal communication and relationships, and dying as a categorical indication of the hospice patient's eligibility for hospice services. In the following discussion, I will distinguish these different uses of the word by referring to the categorical term as *dying*.

At what point do we say that a person is dying? As Tom, Sarah, and I talked about it in the interviews, we often used the term *dying* to refer to the regulations governing hospice services, rather than to a specific course of bodily deterioration. Because hospice services are reimbursed through Medicare, Medicaid, and private insurance—hospice-as-organization must adhere carefully to the criteria for each patient's admission into hospice and the continuation of his or her hospice services (Miller et al., 2000). These criteria are used to determine when a patient is dying so that hospice services are provided to the appropriate patients, and reimbursement funds are spent or conserved according to standardized procedures. By categorizing some people as dying, hospice also tries to ensure that patients are referred early enough for hospice services to do the most good. But dying also refers to a patient's anticipated physical death, which is an inevitable reality toward which all hospice services—including the volunteers's visits—are ultimately directed. Both the anticipated physical death of the patient (dying) and the constructed reimbursable category (*dying*) have tangible effects on the volunteer–patient relationship. In this chapter, Tom's and Sarah's stories about their relationships with their patients were framed by their understanding that their patients did not conform to the *dying* category.

During the training we learned that a patient is admitted to the program when his or her primary care physician and hospice determine that he or she has 6 months or less to live. Medicare beneficiaries have unlimited coverage for hospice care, with two 90-day benefit periods covered by an unlimited number of 60-day periods, for as long as their prognosis does not change (Miller et al., 2000). Hospice admission requirements state that a patient must fit within the dying category to be classified as appropriate (i.e., legally eligible) for hospice services. The volunteers also learned that if a patient begins to improve after he or she enters a hospice program, he or she can be reevaluated and graduate, as had happened with Dorothy several years before, as well as with Sarah's patient by the end of the study. Although we knew that graduating from hospice was a possibility for our patients, we had also internalized the canonical story for a hospice volunteer, which is to visit a patient, to make a difference in his or her life, then to say goodbye to when it is time to go.

For the most part, the volunteers in my study visited patients whose health declined until they died. In one sense, a patient's death gave significance and closure to the volunteer–patient relationship because it meant that the volunteer had been providing companionship and comfort to someone *at the end of life*. According to our construction of hospice and our role as volunteers, this is what we were *supposed* to do. Thus, we appropriated the category of dying to make our role meaningful. When our patients died, we found it comforting to know that we had reached the suitable and expected conclusion to the story. In her first interview, Hannah described how her first patient died soon after she began visiting her, but Hannah saw evidence that she had provided comfort to her patient, and to her patient's family, when she saw them at the nursing home 2 days before her patient died. Hannah said, "Even though I was only able to have two meetings with her, probably one of the best things was being able to share with them [the family] … seeing how grateful they were." Hannah interpreted her experience in terms of the canonical volunteer story, of which the death of her patient was an integral part.

When her patient graduated, Sarah's volunteer story concluded with an acceptable, albeit rare, variation of the canonical ending. However, there were two aspects of Sarah's situation that were highly unusual. First, from the very beginning of her relationship with her patient, Sarah's knowledge of end-of-life care meant that she knew her patient may not fit the category of dying, which in turn meant that her patient might graduate. Several months into volunteering, it was obvious that

Sarah had become quite close to her patient and provided companionship and support during the months that she visited with her. At the same time, Sarah sensed that she was not fulfilling the role of a hospice volunteer because her patient was not dying, and had a strong support network of family, friends, and church.

Sarah's case illustrates how the dying category can affect the volunteer's evaluation of her performance. If we accept the premise of the dying category, it is impossible to be an appropriate, let alone successful, hospice volunteer if one is volunteering for an inappropriate hospice patient. In addition, all the volunteers evaluated their work on the basis of how much they believed a patient was benefiting from the visits. For example, one of the reasons I found my early visits with Dorothy so difficult was because I did not know if I was contributing anything to her life. This violated a tenet of the volunteer–patient relationship story, in which the volunteer is supposed to "make a difference" in the life of the patient and not the other way around—an assumption that I critique at the end of Part IV.

Sarah accurately anticipated her patient's graduation from hospice, but none of the other volunteers were informed if or when their patients's cases were being reviewed. Although hospice did not inform us of any review process, Tom and I conducted our own assessments of our patients' appropriateness, and prepared ourselves for the contingency of having our patients taken off the program. In his second interview, Tom told me he did not believe his patient fit into the dying category, and, furthermore, that there was "no way" he would stop seeing him or reduce the frequency of his visits. In addition to his feelings of attachment, Tom couldn't tolerate the idea that his patient would be left all alone.

Around the same time that I spoke with Tom about his patient, I was also wondering about Dorothy's appropriateness for the hospice program, because her health seemed to have improved rather than deteriorated. I found out later that Dorothy, who had COPD, fit into the same trajectory as Sarah's patient, who had congestive heart failure, because they both had "chronic illness with gradual decline and periodic crises that may result in sudden death" (Bradley et al., 2000, p. 66). Six months into my relationship with Dorothy, I had become accustomed to seeing her every week. I felt close to her and appreciated by her. Although Dorothy, like Sarah's patient, was living at home with family members, I knew that she liked to go out, and I felt that the times we spent together were special for both of us. As strange as it might seem from an outsider's perspective, I disliked the idea that Dorothy could be taken off the hospice program. Although it would mean that Dorothy was no longer dying, it would also mean that hospice expected me to stop seeing her, which was *not* how our story was supposed to end.

When I spoke to Norma, my volunteer coordinator, about my feelings, she gently reminded me that my role was to provide companionship *at the end of life*, and it would be neither appropriate nor helpful to Dorothy for me to continue seeing her once she was no longer in the program. In the same conversation, however, Norma acknowledged that hospice could not dictate what volunteers did on our own time. I often saw Norma go above and beyond in her duties as a coordinator, so I interpreted her comment to mean that I could keep seeing Dorothy, as long as I did not allow my visits to interfere with my official volunteer work. Although I could be mistaken, I did not get the impression that Norma disapproved of the closeness of my relationship with Dorothy or my sense of commitment. Rather, Norma was fulfilling her role as a hospice representative by pointing out how continuing to visit Dorothy could keep her, at least psychologically, in the dying category, as well as overburdening my time so that I would have less to give to another appropriate patient. When hospice suspends its services, the patient can construe this as positive because it signals a return to a more stable state of health; however, the patient may not interpret the loss of his or her volunteer in the same way. For patients like Tom's, the loss of a volunteer compounds the pain of social dying—a concept I explain more fully in Part IV—which may have begun long before the patient was determined to be dying.

At a certain point in our relationships with our patients, our commitment to them went beyond hospice rules and regulations. Our relationships were rewarding to us and we could not just remove ourselves from our patients' lives; it didn't feel right, or appropriate, to do that. Volunteers are not only representatives of hospice-as-organization; we also have our own unique sense of what is right and appropriate in terms of our relationships with patients. Further, Tom and I looked beyond the regulations to the spirit of hospice-as-philosophy, and recognized that our patients were at the end of their lives and we wanted to continue to visit them for as long as they benefitted from our company. Further complicating the volunteer's sense making is the subjective experience of being with a particular patient. Although Sarah's volunteering relationship was very similar to mine—she was visiting a patient in her home, who had a caregiver with her and seemed relatively healthy—she anticipated her patient's graduation from hospice with somewhat different feelings because of unique circumstances with which Sarah had become familiar. Tom felt very strongly about his responsibilities to his patient because of the unique relationship that they had established, and given other circumstances, he might make a different decision about continuing to see his patient. Our perspectives on hospice-as-organization and our role within it changed in response to hospice-as-experienced with our patients. One implication of this is that for volunteers like Tom, who have little ongoing contact with the organization, the relationship rules that emerge through visiting patients override what they understand of hospice rules. One of the greatest strengths of hospice-as-philosophy is the freedom and flexibility that it gives the volunteers regarding our relationships with patients. At the same time, there are many risks associated with establishing a close relationship with a patient who is at the end of life, and sometimes hospice-as-organization is not sufficiently flexible to accommodate what the volunteer believes is the right thing to do.

7

Caring Without Conversation

In the story that concludes chapter 6, when Terry asked me about whether in an emergency she should call 9-1-1 instead of hospice, I faced the issue of whether Terry and Dorothy understood hospice as end-of-life care. Just as Tom was caught off guard when his patient mentioned the priest coming by to give him the last rites, I was not prepared to talk explicitly with Dorothy about her DNR order and what that meant in terms of resuscitation, mostly because we had never spoken of her illness. Until that point, it would be difficult to identify how my interactions with Dorothy differed from those we would share as friends; it was only during the conversation about her wishes regarding artificial respiration and life support that I took on the role of a representative of hospice. Although we could have talked about her death at any time, I left the initiation of that conversation up to her, and as it happened, Dorothy's pronouncement regarding "The Man Upstairs" was the only time we talked explicitly about her illness and death. Despite the stereotype that a meaningful death involves talking through the dying process with hospice patients, Dorothy and I tended to talk about family, the past, and life in general, rather than the details of her health or her feelings about her death. Conversations played a large role in our relationship, but they were not the kinds of conversation many would imagine when thinking about hospice volunteering.

In this chapter, I present stories related to the experience of visiting with someone who can not have a conversation about death or anything else. If my experiences with Dorothy challenged the stereotypes I held regarding communication at the end of life, Emilia's and Chris's experiences made me revise my assumptions about what constitutes meaningful communication in all interpersonal contexts.

EMILIA

Emilia and I meet at a restaurant in our neighborhood. Our original plan was to conduct our interview over dinner and then see a movie. Instead, we end up talking for most of the evening in the restaurant and then in the small garden outside once we finish our meal. I slip easily into an informal and animated conversation with Emilia. By the time of our second meeting, Emilia's first patient has died. I appreciate how open she is about all dimensions of her experiences, particularly the aspects she has found to be uncomfortable or unpleasant.

"I loved my first patient!" Emilia begins. "She was so sweet. Visiting her was tough because she was very confused and it took a while for me to learn to interpret her. But I'm feeling happy because today I sat with my new patient. She has her own room, with furniture. The nursing home is a lot nicer, and it doesn't smell. I was so happy when I found out she could see and she could hear. She learned my name!"

"Your first patient never knew your name?" I ask.

"No, she never did," Emilia replies, shaking her head. "She knew my face but that was all. I can see that hospice is going to be all sorts of experiences. While I was there today with my patient, Susan, a confused lady came to the door and was talking to herself. Susan turned to me and asked, 'What's *she* doing here?' It was almost as if we were friends. It was so comfortable today, and I was happy about that. But it also bothered me because I realized that's not what it's supposed to be about."

I interject. "What? It's not about you being comfortable? But in the last nursing home I remember you had to stand in the hallway all the time, without a chair!" I sense that Emilia feels bad for complaining about the situation at the last nursing home.

"Yeah," Emilia agrees reluctantly. "And there was the deaf lady who used to scream at me all the time. But that's all a part of being in hospice. It's reality. This could happen to me; this could happen to the people I love. My former patient was so sweet, but it was *work*. One time she thought we were in a car. We were in the hallway and she thought her son Lawrence was driving, and she kept saying 'Tell Lawrence to stop! Tell him to turn around! Look at the turkey! This is the wrong way!' She was looking at the wallpaper. I just thought, 'Go along with it.' So I said, 'Miss Palmer, I think we're going the right way.'

"Every visit was worse. The time before last, there was vomit on her pillow. She was in the bed and I tried to help her to eat, but she wanted to lie down and she screamed 'Put me in bed!' It was very hard—hard to see vomit on her pillow."

"So what happened when she died?" I ask.

"The last time," Emilia sighs and shakes her head. "I decided to go see her early. Patrice had called to say I'd better go. Miss Palmer's son and his wife were there. I had tried to call them to introduce myself but they never called me back. Miss Palmer was sleeping peacefully, but it was the *worst* visit because I didn't know what to do when I saw them. I walked in and the son didn't look at me. The daughter-in-law did, though she looked at me like, 'Who the hell are you?' So, I just said, 'I'm Miss Palmer's hospice volunteer. I realize you're spending time with her so I'll come back later. I just wanted to let you know how much I enjoyed meeting Miss Palmer and spending time with her.' The daughter-in-law said, 'Well, don't bother coming anymore because she's dying now.'

"I told myself, 'Okay Emilia, don't judge, because everybody's different. It's the last hour and people say things they wouldn't normally say.'

"Then, the daughter-in-law started talking a little bit. The son never looked at me. She told me Miss Palmer was nearly 100—that's how old she was! And she told me some stories, about all the things she'd done. Then I noticed a little bit of guilt. She said, 'Well, we can't come here that often. We live so far away.' And I said, 'Yes, I understand.' I don't even remember what I said, exactly. It was *extremely* uncomfortable. It was the worst! I didn't even address the son, but she put her hand out, and I put my hand on her shoulder and told her it was good to meet her. Miss Palmer passed away the next day and I sent a card to them.

"I felt like an idiot. Like, shit! What are you supposed to say? I called Patrice and told her these people weren't very nice. Patrice said, 'Yeah, they were kind of weird. They were never friendly.' At least I know it's not me! So, that was my 'final hour.' I was happy to see she was not gasping for breath; she was in a deep sleep. She looked pretty. So, I think it was a happy ending; once a week was enough, though, because it was hard work. With this new patient it's a different type of friendship. She likes to talk, so I let her do her thing."

"Sounds like it was comfortable for you today," I prompt.

"Exactly. But if she started crying to me and saying, 'I don't know what to do,' or 'I'm dying,' that would not be as uncomfortable as that moment with the children of my first patient. I'm not an expert, but because I had that experience of losing my mother, I do understand what it's like. I'm sympathetic, but it's hard for me sometimes to deal with the silent individual who leaves me guessing what they're thinking. I'm working on that. Maybe that's what the problem was with the family—I didn't know them. Maybe if I could have walked in and hugged them it wouldn't have been so uncomfortable. It was too intense."

Emilia pauses for a moment. "I don't know how you're even going to write this. I guess your purpose isn't necessarily to find an answer, right?"

"Right. It's to share all of the stories, the thoughts and lessons that we learned—things that worked and things that didn't. What makes the writing challenging is that there is such a range of experiences."

"Exactly," Emilia agrees. "Even something like the difference in situations and settings. My first nursing home smelled a lot and this one smells a little. I'm more comfortable, and today I smiled a lot. My patient is so cute—I mean, she has sores and one wandering eye, but I just felt a real positive energy. She said she had a good relationship with God. She had four people die of lung cancer in one year; her husband passed away; now she's in a nursing home and some people are not nice to her. I heard her saying all this and she was so sweet. I said, 'Some people are just not very nice; like with me, some nurses here are nice and some aren't.'

"I'm almost relieved because it's like a break right now. I know I will have patients who have a harder time dealing with the fact that this is their time. I think this lady is finding some things hard, but then she'll say, 'God is so good and I can't complain.' It seems so simple. She said, 'I'm in this nursing home because I couldn't take care of myself. I'm so lucky and my neighbors are so good. The person next door used to bring fresh things to me every day. This person still calls me every day, although she can't talk for long.' I was sitting there thinking, 'You're so nice!' It's such a relief to sit with somebody like that."

"So, how long do you get to spend with her?"

"With my first patient, I would spend an average of an hour per week. It sounds horrible, but there was only so much of myself I could put in for a week, and with this lady I can do more. I know Miss Palmer appreciated my visits. We would hold hands. But now I feel I could have done more. Now, I *will* try to do more with this patient."

"You seem to be quite hard on yourself. Don't you think it's important to be realistic about the down sides?" I ask. "You volunteered in a nursing home that smelled bad, and they didn't have a chair for you ...."

"There was vomit on her pillow," Emilia interjects.

"... those things all have an impact on you." I conclude.

"I liked to visit Miss Palmer, but I didn't like her surroundings. I think that's what it was. It was very hard to sit in the hallway with the lady screaming and patients going back and forth. There was no privacy. But, I had to remind myself that I'm in hospice and it could be worse than this. And then with her dementia, it sucks because the nurses don't care and don't have the time to try to understand her. But at least she has dementia and doesn't have to smell the smells—or she transforms all of it into home cooking, or something!

"I never felt sorry for Miss Palmer. She was 99 years old, and although I'm young, I would have a hard time taking care of somebody like that, given my daily activities. So, I said, 'This is reasonable.' People say, 'Oh my God, how do you do hospice?' And I say, 'First of all, I'm new and I don't know how I do it, but it can't be worse than dealing with little kids who are being abused or battered wives.' I cried when Miss Palmer died just because sometimes something is so good that I get emotional. I thought, 'This is so quick and good, everything is going to be okay.' But I don't think I'll really know what it's like to be in hospice until I'm dealing with someone who's unfairly dying. I think it would be tough if somebody turned to me and said, 'Oh my God, I'm leaving my family. I'm 50. I have a couple of kids. Why me?'

"I think different volunteers are cut out for different things. When Miss Palmer died, I didn't want to go back to that nursing home yet. I thought the nurses were kind of rude. I tried to be gentle and nice, but I realized you can't be. I'd say, 'Could you please help me to lift Miss Palmer?' They'd say, 'Oh, honey, she's so small you could do it yourself.' I'd have to say, 'No, actually, I can't. I'm from hospice and I'm not allowed to.' I didn't know how to deal with it! The nursing homes are tough that way."

I observe, "I'm visiting my patient in her home and I feel protective of her, too. Anything that makes her feel uncomfortable ...."

"Like, neglect?" Emilia interjects.

"No, not neglect," I clarify. "Her relationship with her daughter is great. Terry moved so she could take care of Dorothy, but she doesn't spend as much time at home as she used to. Dorothy makes indirect comments about that, but then I remind myself that I'm only getting one person's story." I think about the role of the nursing home staff—or nurses—as they are referred to in these interviews, regardless of their actual titles or functions. I'm not really getting *their* side of the story, though I'm sure a lot of it has to do with being understaffed and underappreciated.

"Also," Emilia adds, "we're going into that situation as hospice, not family. But when it was my mother, there was a little bit of denial—this was *my Mom*: I didn't know she was terminal. Although I should have known—duh!"

"But how could you know if you'd never seen it before?"

"I knew she was really sick, but I had my daily life. New Year's week, my Mom was visiting and my sister was dating a guy and he really wanted to take her out. Mom said, 'Why don't you stay at home?' and my sister said, 'No. I'll be back later.' My mother was really upset. Maybe my mother knew it was her last New Year's Eve. Now we look back and think, 'We should have done this; we should have done that.' Sometimes I wonder, if I could go back knowing what I know today but not knowing that my mom was sick, would that have changed anything? Maybe a little bit, but I'd still spend time with my boyfriend; I'd still go out, because you have to survive. So, from my perspective, we as volunteers may be focused on death and dying, but Dorothy's daughter may not be looking on her as dying at all.

"But the reason I mentioned neglect, my patient Susan has a nice room and a nice view, but she's there *all day long*. She says she sits there and she *thinks*. I can see why some people would start complaining. That would be me. 'You don't spend enough time with me. These people are neglecting me!'

"I walked in on this woman by accident today, thinking it was my patient, and she was asking me for all these things: 'Can you take me to the potty? Can you get me some cookies?' Not that she was imposing, but in contrast, my hospice patient kept asking me, 'Am I taking up too much of your time?'"

"Well," I respond, "it sounds like survival to me. If that other woman has been in the nursing home for a while, then she's probably learned to take every opportunity to get what she needs."

"But don't you think it's weird how people are so different—that we react so differently to all these things? That's why I know your research .... I was thinking, 'She has to listen to these interviews twice. How is she going to put this down?'"

"Twice!" I exclaim. "Oh, much more than that."

"Really?"

"Oh, yeah. By the time I write this up, I will have listened to these five or six times, plus all the times I'll read the transcripts. But we're talking about things that are hard to pin down; that's why it's important to do this research. This is not something you can understand through a survey or getting people to check off the boxes. It's hard to articulate how you learn to be with people who are dying."

Emilia and I shift our conversation away from hospice and continue talking well into the night. Despite her "complaints," Emilia seems to have adapted to volunteering in the nursing home. When Emilia and I first spoke, I felt a little concerned about how her recent experience of losing her mother might affect her feelings about her patient's death. However, she took the death of her first patient in stride, irrespective of the cold reception she got from her patient's family. I note that Emilia constructs the stories of her mother's and her patient's deaths very differently, not only because the relationships were different in each case, but also because she has a sense that some deaths are "fair," or constitute "happy endings," and others are not. I also note that Emilia already perceives herself as able to "do more" for her new patient because they will be able to have a conversation together. Yet, it also appears that Emilia was the only person visiting Miss Palmer in the nursing home. Perhaps the absence of a reciprocal relationship has made it difficult for Emilia to have a sense of her contribution to Miss Palmer's life, and also easier for her to let Miss Palmer go and embrace a new patient.

Because Emilia seems so unperturbed regarding Miss Palmer's death, I begin to wonder how I will react to Dorothy's death. Unlike Emilia's patient, Dorothy is not dying of old age; instead, a disease caused by smoking has shortened her life. Dorothy is in her late 70s, and since she lost her husband, her ability to drive, and her health, her world has become confined accordingly. Although Dorothy's world and her ability to interact may continue to diminish, I feel myself growing closer to her and realize how much she has to share with me and her family. I wonder what circumstances would allow me to frame her death as "fair."

CHRIS

Chris and I meet on campus for our second interview. From an earlier phone conversation, I know that Chris has been seeing a patient for about 3 months, so I ask him to go back to the beginning and talk about meeting his patient at the nursing home.

"Well, Patrice called me, and she explained this location as a place that they couldn't get anybody else to go. She said people felt unsafe in the environment. It's in a nice community, but some may think there are bad elements there. That probably comes from not being familiar with the area. But, the way that Patrice put it, if I didn't go there, nobody would."

"And how could you say no to that?" I ask. It was only later that I wondered why Patrice decided to recruit Chris for this assignment. Was it because he was an experienced, 40-year-old man, or because he was African American, or both? When I asked Chris about it, he felt that both factors had played a part, and also his enthusiasm.

"I took the challenge!" Chris chuckles. "Well, I could have said no for the same reasons that everybody else did. If they don't feel safe then I don't want to go there! I will generally take a challenge like that, though. Through my work as a funeral director, I knew the nursing home that she was talking about, so I didn't have any problems. The patient that I'm seeing, he doesn't talk to me. I don't know if I'm doing him any real good because we don't communicate. But I may be doing some good for hospice because at least I'm able to check up on him, see that he's doing okay, and report that. Patrice said recently, 'If you don't feel comfortable with this, then you can get out of it.' And I said, 'No, I think I can do some good.' I couldn't communicate with him but at least somebody's going to see about him, you know? If I didn't go then nobody would, and that was the worst thought for me."

It seems to me that hospice has a higher purpose for Chris's visits. I ask, "You're trying to establish the safety of this nursing home so that other volunteers will go there, right?"

"Right," Chris affirms. "Because from what Patrice was saying, I think they may need some other volunteers to come in. I guess you could say I'm building a track record for the nursing home. Patrice said she would like me to tell other volunteers that there's nothing at all to worry about as far as safety. The first time I went, I was wondering what they were afraid of. By the time I left, I didn't see anything that they needed to worry about."

"What's your patient like?"

"I know my patient is terminal because he's a hospice patient, but he doesn't look terminal. He's kind of cool. He enjoys sitting on the patio and he just stays to himself most of the time. I always ask the nurses how he's doing. They told me that he didn't bother anybody and didn't cause any trouble. But the time that I told you about—when he bopped somebody on the ear—that was the first time I had any report that he was a mischievous type of individual. So that let me know that there may be things going on that the nurses don't know about. He knew exactly what he was doing because when he went and sat down, he smiled at me."

Chris had described this incident to me over the phone. For reasons that Chris was unable to determine, his patient had walked over to a fellow resident, flicked the man on the ear with a force that made the man yelp, then returned to his seat next to Chris.

"He didn't explain, though, why he thumped this person in the ear?"

"No, he never talked. The only sign he gives is when he wants a cigarette; he'll gesture like he's putting a cigarette in his mouth. And if he wants coffee, he might actually say coffee."

"Why doesn't he talk?" I probe.

Chris explains, "Patrice said he may not be talking to me because he doesn't know me and because of his mental state. Each time I come back, he may not recall ever having seen me. I don't know. He looks like he remembers me, though. When he looks at me, something tells me that he's recognized me."

"So, tell me again about the first time that you went there. You knew the nursing home, so that was familiar to you, and then what happened?"

"Well, the first time, he was in the dining room eating. He was at a round table with other patients. I sat there and tried to get some conversation going and he looked at me like, 'Who is this guy?' He didn't say anything. I guess, under the circumstances, if he was taking in *anything*, he might have been a little apprehensive about the situation. I had on my hospice badge, and he may have seen that as a symbol of authority. I don't know if he could read it, or knew what it was. I'm still trying to figure it all out myself."

"So, how long did you spend there? I think I remember you said ...."

"About 30 minutes," Chris responds.

"Not too long," I observe.

"No, not too long. Because I talk, but he doesn't say anything."

"What do you talk about?"

"I ask him how his day goes and how does his week go, but I don't get any response. I think over the next few weeks I'll try to take him some magazines. I have a little more time and I'll see if it stimulates him, interests him, or maybe causes him to come more alive. That may create more of a connection between us. We'll see. I don't know what else—do you have any ideas of what I could take in there?"

"No," I respond. "I was just thinking that if you could get a little more information about him, his life, what he used to do."

"I'm not sure they have it," Chris shakes his head a little.

"Right." I remember that this man is completely alone and does not speak. "I guess you could start with magazines and see if one thing in particular interests him, then you could go from there. Do you know if he does anything on his own?"

"Other than smoking, eating, and sitting alone, I don't think he does too much more than that, really. Now, I think he has a pretty adult mind. You know how sometimes when people get older they like something that a child might enjoy? I don't think he would enjoy that. I think he has too much of an adult mind."

"Yeah." I agree. "For some reason I had that impression, too. Because all the other things I was thinking about, like clay, or drawing, or stuff like that ...."

"I don't think it would intrigue him at all," Chris chuckles.

"Somehow, with someone who smokes and drinks coffee, I don't see them enjoying puzzles or Legos or toys." It occurs to me that Chris and I may also be trying to avoid treating an older person as if he were a child. It can be a common mistake to equate advanced age, especially when accompanied by Alzheimer's or dementia, with infancy, and potentially strip a person of his or her dignity in the process.

"Do you know if he talks to other people?" I venture.

"No, I don't," Chris shakes his head. "The nurses tell me that the only thing he does is what I told you: to let his needs be known. Now, a few weeks ago, they said he tried to leave the nursing home, so they've put him in a secure section and I have to be buzzed into that section now. They said he just tried to leave."

"So, you go, and he doesn't say anything, and you chat with him ...." I trail off.

"Sometimes, when we're out on the patio, it feels good to me to just sit for a while because I've been running all day. I just sit there and he sits there. He never tries to get away from me. You know, sometimes he looks me in the eye and makes eye contact, so I feel he's communicating at the level of 'I know you're here.' He's not ignoring me."

"Do you have any idea of who you are to him? You said you think he recognizes you when you arrive."

"Yeah, he recognizes me," Chris affirms. "He looks at me, and I can't prove it, but for some reason, I think that he recognizes me. Does he know who I am to him? I doubt it."

"So, what are you getting out of it?" I ask.

"I'm wondering!" Chris smiles and shakes his head, indicating his doubts. "I've thought about that and I don't believe I know, but maybe at some point I'll discover some way to make it more meaningful. Maybe I'll learn how to deal with people who don't talk to me."

I agree. "It's important that we know how to respond to people who don't talk back or converse with us. There are a lot of older people who reach that point and we've got to be able to care *for* them and care *about* them, and not make that care contingent upon their ability to have a conversation. I think for me the hardest thing would be to volunteer with somebody like that." I think about the struggles I had in the early days with Dorothy. Although she could both converse and get around, it was still difficult for me to just be with her. If I couldn't talk with someone, I think I'd find it even harder to establish that level of comfort. Like Chris, I wouldn't know where to begin.

"You could call me and I'll let you know," Chris laughs. "I'll give you my notes on this patient."

"Well, Emilia, too." I add. "She said that was the one kind of patient she didn't want to visit; she wanted someone she could talk to. Then she got to the nursing home and her lady was, 'Where's Lawrence? I'm waiting for Lawrence. Where's Beth?' I think she was an Alzheimer's patient and Emilia said they did the same thing every time she arrived. The woman never recognized her, but Emilia would wheel her around, and they would go and look for Beth and Lawrence, this woman's children. Emilia said, 'We're always doing something, but there's nothing *meaningful* about the interaction.' She did believe that it made a difference that she was there. It made me realize that, at some point, we all have to understand for ourselves how and why this volunteering is a good thing to do."

"I think it's always a good thing to do," Chris agrees. "We don't have all the answers; we're there to do whatever we can and that's all. I know I would never be able to cure anybody of anything, but they'll be there, their condition will get worse, and they'll move on. While they're alive, we can give them something. I'll just have to continue to go, and I may learn how to make the best of a situation where a person doesn't talk to you. But I like that, because I think once you've experienced the roughest situation that there is, then everything else seems easy!"

Chris adds, "And another thing—not that I think the nurses neglect the patients—but by showing up every now and then, that will sort of encourage the nurses to give him the proper attention. And that's with anything. They say if you visit your child at school, the teachers will probably give that child more attention. So that may help, too."

"One thing you talked about in the last interview was the value of human contact. How does that idea fit into this context with this particular patient?"

Chris responds thoughtfully, "I think it's very important in this situation. The nurses tell him when it's time to go to bed, time to eat, time to get up. That's not the kind of human contact that is sufficient. When I go to see him, I sit close to him, to let him know that I am there if he wants to say something, and I do try to talk to him. I don't get any answer, but he looks at me."

"I remember someone telling a story about visiting their nursing home patient, and this patient was obviously proud to be having a visitor," I observe.

"That's nice. I would like that to be true," Chris smiles.

I elaborate. "Because there's somebody coming to visit on a regular basis, that sends a message to the patient about his worth as a human being."

"And to the nursing staff as well. This is a county facility for people who get help from the government, for people of 'very little means,' I think was how Patrice put it. I'm sure some had a pretty good life when they were younger, and they just ended up in those situations."

The idea depresses me. "It just seems so sad to me that people would end up alone."

"There are a lot of those types of situations," Chris replies. "Growing old is probably the worst thing that can happen to a lot of people. You get to grow old and you get cast aside."

"It sounds like you're going to continue to see this patient," I prompt.

"Yes," Chris agrees. "Like I said, I don't know if he's getting anything out of my visits, but I'll continue if it's of any benefit to hospice that I continue to report what I see. The biggest challenge was the other day when I started having doubts about what I've really accomplished, but now that I've crossed that phase, it doesn't bother me. Other than that the biggest thing that bothers me is seeing humans kind of wasting away. I think, 'This is no way for them to spend the last days of their life. You know?'"

"What have you found to be the best thing about volunteering?"

"The best thing is, I would say, being part of something very good. If I'm feeling down, I can always say, 'Well, I'm trying to make things a little bit better for someone.' Then I get to come and talk to you about the experience, and that's a very good part of it." Chris grins.

"I'm very glad," I smile back. What a charmer!

Although Chris had very little to report in terms of his interaction with his patient, I start to reflect upon this interview and why it was difficult for me to identify with Chris's patient. Chris struggled to establish a basis for his relationship with this particular person, because he got none of the cues that we rely on to enter another person's world. Even though Emilia's patient had dementia, Emilia was able to listen for clues that revealed her patient's experience, and thus respond to her patient's reality. In contrast, Chris received very little information from his patient about anything, and so was left guessing about what his patient was experiencing and how to respond personally to him. Perhaps hardest of all, Chris didn't know whether he made any difference in the patient's life, so rather than continuing to look for confirmation from his patient, he established the meaning of this volunteering experience for himself. Chris recognized the value of being present and caring about all types of people who are approaching the end of their lives, not only those who are able to interact in the ways that we most value in our culture.

ANOTHER "SPELL"

When I arrive at Dorothy's apartment today, she is having one of her "spells," as Terry calls them. I am glad that Terry is home this time, because Dorothy's confusion is much worse. As I greet Dorothy and take her hand, Dorothy smiles warmly, but she also seems distracted and confused about who I am. She calls me Ruth, and Terry explains that Ruth is one of Dorothy's sisters. I don't know what to do.

Dorothy strings words together with an intonation that mirrors normal speech, but the words themselves do not make sense. At one point, it seems that she is trying to tell me something about Terry, but she keeps saying "Tuesday." From the depths of my memory one word emerges as clear and evident as Dorothy's words are cloudy and evasive—aphasia. I know that it is the term given to a language impairment that affects speech production or comprehension, but now I am confronted with its manifestation in someone I care about. It scares me. I am awed that Terry is so calm, carefully watching and listening to her mother, seemingly free of anxiety.

Terry meets my wide eyes with a gentle nod and reports, "She does this from time to time. I wish I knew how to predict it, but I don't. It usually happens in the morning, so it might have something to do with her oxygen during the night, but who knows. It will probably pass pretty soon. Why don't I get you a cup of coffee?"

I didn't know that this had been happening regularly. I sit in my spot on the sofa and try to interact with Dorothy, but she is making very little sense. I want to cry. I'm afraid that this change might be permanent, and I realize that I'm not ready for Dorothy to leave.

After about 45 minutes, Dorothy's speech is more coherent, and after an hour, she will not even acknowledge that anything was wrong.

We enjoy a quiet visit at home with Terry, sitting out in the breezeway. I drive home and immediately call LifePath. I wait for Jackie, Dorothy's nurse, to get back to me. Three hours later, Jackie is able to return my call, and I tell her about what happened that morning. I ask her for information about the cause of Dorothy's confusion, so I can share it with Terry next week.

"We'll probably never know," Jackie replies. "It could be oxygen deprivation, it could be tiny strokes. But you have to realize, Elissa, that Dorothy is very sick. She is in a lot of denial about her illness, but don't be fooled."

"But she hardly ever uses her oxygen during our visits," I reply. "She doesn't cough as much as she used to. She seems to be getting better, not worse."

"You need to be prepared," Jackie responds, firmly. "That's a trick of this disease. It can be unpredictable. And it certainly doesn't help that Dorothy won't acknowledge that she's sick. I've known Dorothy for a long time, and I can tell you now, if you hadn't told me about this, and if Terry happened to be working during my next visit, Dorothy would never have told me that this happened today."

I thank Jackie for calling back, and she says, "Call me any time. I don't want you to be confused about what's going on here."

As we end our phone call, I think about all the positive signs that I see in Dorothy every time I visit, and compare that to what Jackie has told me about Dorothy's condition. The two images don't add up for me. I want to believe that Dorothy is telling the truth whenever she says, "I'm fine." At the same time, I know that she is a hospice patient, and hospice patients are, by definition, terminally ill.

I feel my stomach turn itself inside out as I remember sitting with Dorothy today. I was so afraid that she would remain confused and not get better. Perhaps Jackie is right when she says I need to be prepared, because I certainly don't feel prepared right now. I know that the idea of visiting Dorothy will be radically different if she does suffer a stroke and can no longer speak to me. I have come to rely on our ritual of going out to eat lunch together and hanging out in the breezeway before and after our outings. Even the silences that used to be so awkward and difficult for me have taken on a different quality after so many hours of conversation. I don't know if I could adjust to visits like those that Chris shares with his patient, not knowing if he is communicating with a conscious person or not.

On the other hand, what if Jackie is wrong and Dorothy does get better and she "graduates" again? Even in that very happy situation, I would be asked to stop seeing her as a patient, and that idea makes me feel awful. I guess, deep down, I know that I wouldn't stop seeing Dorothy just because she graduated from hospice. I would, like Tom, keep seeing her as a friend, despite the regulations. With that insight, I realize that I would also continue to see Dorothy if her condition changes for the worse; I would find some other way to be with her and bring her happiness. She would need my company no less then than if she got better and graduated. I would just need to learn from Chris and Emilia and be prepared to improvise, potentially to get it "wrong," and to persevere with my commitment to be there for Dorothy.

REFLECTIONS: ASSUMPTIONS ABOUT THE VALUE OF "TALK" IN HOSPICE

I begin this reflection by returning to an issue I introduced in chapter 2, specifically, Seale's (1998) contention that hospice is overly reliant on discourse or "talk" in the ways that it approaches finding meaning at the end of life. Bradshaw (1996) makes a similar observation, suggesting that modern or psychosocial approaches "presume verbal activity, counseling, talking, self-expression; 'getting in touch with feelings' by expressing them" (p. 414). Bradshaw further suggests that what is lost is the ability to just *be* with the patient and family. From the volunteers' stories and my own experience, I resist the notion that the hospice philosophy of "the good death" overemphasizes the patient's ability to talk through his or her experience of death (Lawton, 2000; Seale, 1998, Walter, 1994). This criticism is directed at hospice-as-philosophy, and I agree that some texts (Byock, 1997; Callanan & Kelley, 1992) construct hospice from a perspective that suggests a psychological, rather than a social, understanding of hospice work. However, speaking at the level of hospice-as-experienced, the stories in this book suggest that the daily work of volunteering does not privilege conversations over other kinds of "being with" and understanding hospice patients.

The LifePath Hospice training emphasized that volunteers should provide companionship and support to patients; also, that they should *not* initiate discussions about death and dying with their patients. The volunteers in this study entered relationships with their patients assuming that they should find ways to help patients through the process of dying, but without talking specifically about dying. Notwithstanding the training, it was natural for some of us to assume conversation to be the primary means through which we could achieve our purpose as hospice volunteers. Because Western culture tends to conflate processes of cognition, communication, and understanding (Gergen, 1994), it may be hard to resist the commonly held assumption that the only way to "come to terms" with something is to understand it, which implies thinking about it, which in turn implies talking about it (Jourard, 1971).

The media contribute somewhat to this premise by representing the dying process as one in which people actively reflect on the meaning of their lives and share their thoughts and feelings with others. The PBS documentary series *On Our Own Terms* (Public Affairs Television, 2000) presented the deaths of a variety of people who were, without exception, self-reflexive and highly articulate about illness, spirituality, and their own deaths. Moreover, during the volunteer training we viewed a video of Morrie Schwartz on *Nightline*, during which he spoke openly about his illness and death. Unwittingly, this video may have contributed to our fantasy of what discussions about dying would be like with our patients, and how we would know when they had "come to terms" with their deaths.

As the stories in this book demonstrate, however, once we met our patients and began the experience of visiting with them, very little of our interaction focused specifically on dying. In the first round of interviews, I discussed with Hannah and Tom how unprepared we felt when we graduated from the training, and part of the reason for this was that the hospice training did not tell us what would occur during interactions with patients. Sarah said that she appreciated this aspect of the training: "They didn't try to tell you how to handle it. They were honest in saying you have to go in there and see what happens." The nondirective approach of the training translated into a nondirective approach by the volunteers in their relationships—we had to learn to wait and see what emerged from our interactions. In my relationship with Dorothy, for several weeks it seemed as though nothing happened, and I called Norma because I thought Dorothy was going to fire me. However, something *was* happening between Dorothy and me, and my error was thinking that there had to be some kind of direct effort on my part to *do* something *for* Dorothy.

When I complained to Shyanne about my perceived failure as a volunteer, she shared a perspective that helped me to revise my assumptions about communicating with my patient, and helped me to consider "just being" with someone as a perfectly legitimate response:

"I think in our society we get so used to being these little human doings .... But you're a human being. And that word *being* is what we give to our patients .... Sometimes they don't even need us to give them any pearls of wisdom or to say anything: just a nod of the head or a smile or holding their hand."

As Shyanne's statement suggests, *being with* our patients often meant being comfortable with silence. I remember feeling thrilled the day I realized that Dorothy and I had been sitting together for several minutes, and for the first time, I hadn't felt compelled to fill the silence. With his first patient, Tom said he found the silence challenging, but recognized its value:

> "I felt the need to keep the conversation going, and with her not contributing the only thing I could really talk about was me .... But I remembered Patrice saying it's fine just to sit there and not say a word. So I said, "Do you want me to leave? Because you look really tired." And she said, "No, I'm just tired. But I want you to stay." So I just sat there looking at her and every now and then she would open her eyes to see if I was still there."

One of the things that Tom and I had to overcome was our sense of self-consciousness, which is an expected part of any early interaction between strangers (Berger & Calabrese, 1975). However, we also had the added constraint of being overly conscious of our role as hospice volunteers, and not yet sure of what was the right thing to do. By the second round of interviews, our relationships with our patients had moved from an impersonal to a more personal level, and we felt more comfortable and less self-conscious about our communication.

Dorothy and I did not talk about her illness and approaching death; perhaps it was "denial," as Jackie suggested to me, or perhaps it was simply that she did not wish to spend our time together talking about death. As the stories in this chapter illustrate, sometimes there are practical reasons why a volunteer is not able to talk explicitly with a patient about death. Emilia's patient had dementia, and it was soon apparent that her patient did not always know where she was or that she was in the hospice program. Emilia said, "I think I keep her physically and mentally active. I think I'm helping, but in terms of dealing with death? I don't even think she realizes." Emilia also emphasized how much happier and more comfortable she felt with her new patient because she could have a conversation with her. Given that hospice-as-organization assigns volunteers to patients who can not speak as well as those that do, part of the work of the volunteer is to make sense of what we provide to patients beyond conversation and interaction.

Chris's story stands out from the others because it does not appear to fit any of the aspects of the canonical story for hospice volunteers. Like others, Chris told me that his patient "didn't look terminal," and he questioned whether his patient was actually dying, just as Tom and I had with our patients. Also, because Chris's patient did not communicate with him verbally at all, it was difficult for Chris to know how, when, or if he was contributing to his patient's quality of life. To some extent, all of the volunteers had to generate their own story about the meaning of their relationships with patients and how they were "making a difference." Even Emilia's patient, who had Alzheimer's, gave signs that she liked to see Emilia and enjoyed her company. In contrast, Chris struggled to understand the meaning of his interactions with his patient, but ultimately constructed a story that established the value of what he was doing every week.

In our first interview, Chris said, "Human contact, especially when you're getting older, is so important because that's what keeps the minds of seniors active." He also wanted to know how hospice decides to release someone, particularly if he or she still needs the human contact that hospice provides. He elaborated on this idea by saying, "Human contact is extremely valuable, and you can't replace that with anything else. It keeps people alive. I guess without human contact, it would be like that situation where they say, 'If a tree falls in the forest ....' You would have someone alive, but there's no other human contact, so are they really alive? Are they experiencing life?" Chris made these observations before he had met his first patient, and once he started visiting his patient—who didn't communicate with him—this philosophy of "human contact" became a key element in Chris's construction of his role in this patient's life.

In Chris's second interview, he suggested that, at the very least, visiting his patient at the nursing home let the staff know that someone cared about him, so they would not neglect him. In our discussion, we interpreted human contact as a way to communicate a person's value, which is why we were distressed by the idea that people are sometimes cast aside and left to die alone, particularly in nursing homes. This theme of "being all alone" runs through the interviews in two ways; volunteers are motivated to visit patients to ensure that they are "not alone" at the end of their lives, and patients (such as Shyanne's) say that "being alone" is the most frightening aspect of their anticipated death. Because Hannah herself had considered the distressing possibility that she might be alone at the end of her life, she identified with her first patient because she was essentially alone. The volunteers' discourse reveals the conviction that human contact is an antidote to the worst aspect of dying—being alone or lonely. This belief runs deep into the heart of what motivates volunteers to enter relationships with patients and to *continue these relationships* even if the patients cannot communicate that they are aware of the contact.

8

Being Together, Letting Go

SEPTEMBER 11, 2001

It has been a day of terror that we will never forget. It is late afternoon when I call Terry.

"Terry, it's Elissa," I say.

"Hi, honey," Terry replies. "How are you doing?"

"I'm okay," I reply, "It's been a crazy day. I can hardly believe all this is happening."

"I know, I know," Terry replies in a soothing voice. "Did you have anybody up there in New York or D.C.?"

"Yes," I reply, "But we've been in touch with everyone. And I've called my parents in Australia, so they know what's going on. I was worried about Len, though. Where is he right now? Have you been in touch with him?"

"He's in South Carolina," Terry replies. "He's fine. Everybody's fine."

"I'm so glad," I say. "I was calling because tomorrow is supposed to be my visit with Dorothy. How is she doing?"

"Mom's doing great," Terry replies. "Do you want to talk to her?"

"Sure," I reply, and then wait for Dorothy's voice on the other end of the line. "Hi, Dorothy, how are you doing?"

"I'm fine, honey," Dorothy responds.

"What a terrible day!" I exclaim, not sure what else to say.

"It's sure crazy," Dorothy replies. "You can't get anything on the television except this crazy business. Everyone seems to forget that we've been through all this before. I don't understand why they have to keep talking about it all the time."

I'm struck silent for a moment by Dorothy's apparent nonchalance. It probably is very different for her. I recall that Stan survived two wars, and then they lost their son in Vietnam. Part of me is dumb-founded that she appears completely insensitive to the political impli-cations of today's events, let alone the tragedy that has occurred for thousands of people. And yet, another part of me is comforted that Dorothy sees this as a remote occurrence, in another part of the world, which has not touched her personally, and so she refuses to let it shake her spirit.

I respond, "I guess it's just scary to some of us because we've never seen anything like this before, Dorothy. It feels like everything's upside down."

"Well," Dorothy pauses for a moment and then says, "I'm still here. You're still here. Life goes on."

"I suppose you're right," I reply.

"Will we see you tomorrow then?" Dorothy asks.

"Of course, I'm looking forward to it. I'll see you around 10:30."

"10:30 or 11," Dorothy replies, "Whichever is better for you."

I suddenly feel tears in my eyes and my throat begins to tighten. I say, "Okay, Dorothy, I'll see you tomorrow morning. Say goodbye to Terry for me."

"I will, honey," Dorothy replies. "Goodbye."

I've cried a lot today, and I start to cry again. This time, I am crying be-cause in these few minutes talking to Dorothy, I realize that her world has not changed. In the midst of the chaos and grief, of wondering if I'll ever get home to see my family again, of fearing that there will be more violence, these moments of talking to Dorothy were the same as they've ever been, normal, and comforting. I can hardly wait to arrive at Doro-thy's apartment, to cocoon myself in her world, if only for a couple of hours. I know I will feel safe.

DOROTHY'S BIRTHDAY

There is a pleasant change in the weather as September gives way to Oc-tober. It is Dorothy's birthday today; she is 78 years old. Having checked the night before with Terry, I surprise Dorothy by arriving on a nonvisiting day with a bunch of flowers and some cupcakes. Dorothy shows off the new velour running suit that Terry gave her, which is both sporty and a terribly feminine shade of pink. I note that someone, prob-ably Leslie, has painted Dorothy's nails and toenails. Dorothy uses this as an opportunity to point out what a tomboy she was as a child, never interested in wearing "ribbons and frills." She hunts around for an al-bum and soon we are peering at a black and white photo of a girl, 10 or 11 years old, wearing a pale dress with a low sash, and a floppy bow holding back a dark pageboy haircut. This is Dorothy of long ago, glowering darkly at the photographer, ready to kill. "Pretty little thing, wasn't I?" Dorothy says sarcastically, rolling her eyes.

"Actually," I say, "You are beautiful." The photograph and the vicious expression of the girl in it do not conceal her delicate features and amazing eyes.

"Like a pig in a petticoat," Dorothy declares, and everyone laughs. "My father made me wear that silly getup."

Terry leans in and kisses her mother warmly on the cheek. "How about some coffee and a cupcake Mom?"

"Let's all have some," Dorothy responds.

I'm pleased to be included in the festivities, and glad that Dorothy is permitting us to make a fuss of her. Terry will be taking Dorothy on a trip this weekend to visit Terry's sister, Connie, and her husband, Chuck, who live in a suburb of Miami. I'm happy that Dorothy is able to travel and that she is spending time with her family. This trip also means that Terry will have a vacation for the first time since I met her.

HANNAH

Hannah and I meet at the same coffee shop as before, but this time on a Saturday morning. We sit at a small table against the wall, which provides a sense of privacy, even though we are surrounded by a crowd of patrons clamoring for their morning lattes and cappuccinos.

"You visited your first patient only very briefly before she passed away," I begin. "Could you catch me up on what's happened since then?"

"Sure," Hannah replies, smiling. "I have a new patient; she is actually very healthy, although obviously she has a terminal diagnosis. She's in her early 90s, a very petite woman, and such a pleasure! I've been with her for 3 months already. Her family visits her often, so she's not alone. I think her biggest adjustment was moving to a nursing home. Until recently she was driving and doing everything on her own, but she has poor vision. It's very frustrating for her. For the first month, we talked about why she had to come to the nursing home—but now we don't talk about it as much, and she's settling in. She's absolutely great! She feels God has been so kind to her that God's plan for her is fine. We don't focus on any of the issues we discussed in hospice training. Instead, we talk about whatever she wants, which sometimes is nothing."

I smile and ask a little facetiously, "You don't feel like you're helping her with her existential questions?"

Hannah smiles and shakes her head, "Not at *all*. She even introduces me to people as her hospice volunteer. You know how we wear our ID badges but no one is supposed to know why we're there? Well, I go on Saturdays and we play bingo and she introduces me to everybody as a hospice volunteer, so I really feel that she's accepted what's going to happen."

"It sounds like you've developed a great relationship with this lady," I observe.

"I have," Hannah replies, smiling warmly. "I think even more so because my mother works there as well. Every time Miss Elliott sees my mother she asks about me. When I leave, she gives me a big hug and thanks me for coming, and tells me she loves me. So she's becoming more than a patient. We talk a lot about faith, which I think is so important, and I learn a lot from her. Sometimes, I think I may be getting too attached, because when she passes I know that I'll feel much more than I expected to."

"I've wondered the same thing about my patient."

"You've spent a long time with her," Hannah smiles and nods.

"I've been with her since February. At one point, I was afraid that she might be taken off the program, but there's been some deterioration in her condition, so I know I'll continue to see her. But how do we know if we're getting *too* attached?"

"I don't," Hannah responds shaking her head. "On my way here to the interview, I thought I might call Patrice to ask about that. I know we're supposed to focus on *them*, but Miss Elliott has this way of turning our conversations around to *me*. It's as if she doesn't want to talk about herself, perhaps because she's really content, and I think that's brought me even closer to her. It can't be *bad* to get close, but I don't want to suffer as a result."

"Particularly not to the point where you don't want to volunteer again," I agree.

"Exactly. I don't know how the people at hospice do it."

"The volunteers spend more time with the patients than any of the other hospice workers," I suggest. "Our 'job' is essentially to have a relationship, whereas the others provide services and facilitate care. This project fascinates me because I'm beginning to understand that the volunteers are like friends who arrive almost from nowhere, and we try to have a positive impact. How do you keep the reins on that?"

"I don't think you can," Hannah replies. "We want to have an effect on their lives, and we want them to have an effect on ours, and obviously they *are*, because we're thinking, 'This is really going to be painful when this person leaves.' As I think about it now, I feel like I'm going to cry because I don't want anything to happen to her!"

"I understand. For a while I felt very elevated and spiritual about the 'Circle of Life,' and that idea that 'I'm being here with Dorothy in the time that she has.' I guess I felt prepared. But as time went on, I got used to our visits, and it became part of my life to be in her life."

Hannah continues, "You think you prepare *them* for the moment when they pass, but in reality, you have to prepare you for the moment when they pass."

"Right! One thing I believe is that we communicate with our patients *as people*, not as *dying* people. We relate to them as living, vital human beings, who can teach us something and who are part of our daily life. But what happens if we really start to forget they're dying?"

Hannah agrees, enthusiastically. "That's what I mean! I almost feel selfish because I shouldn't be thinking about what I'll feel when she passes—because I'm there for *her*. At the same time, having lost people who are close to me, I know how much it can hurt. It's that feeling that scares me so much.

"I'm also constantly pressed for time and I wish that I could spend more time with her. I'm going to miss being with her, talking with her. I'll miss her stories about the Grand Canyon and her travels," Hannah smiles. "She's so descriptive and she's so kind and so affectionate. She gives me a hug when she leaves. She totally initiated that."

I notice that Hannah unconsciously said, 'She gives me a hug when *she* leaves,' instead of 'when I leave.' Perhaps this slip reveals how much her patient's death is preying on her mind.

"How long do you spend with her?" I ask.

"I spend about an hour and a half each time."

"And you do that twice a week?"

"About twice a week. Sometimes three times a week. We play bingo, but we also interact a lot. I'll ask her, 'How is your roommate doing?' And she'll say, 'Great! Last night I had to use the restroom, and she wasn't covered, so I covered her up.' She's in her early 90s and the lady next to her is in her 60s! She's so motherly. Every time I walk in, she asks, 'Are you hungry? I have plenty of cookies. I'll give you some.' Although I only spend 3 or 4 hours with her a week, I feel as if we spend much more time together."

I think about how this relationship has surprised Hannah; it does seem unusually close.

I observe, "Perhaps as volunteers we're prepared to care about the patient, but the big surprise comes when they start caring about us."

"Right. So, the fact that she finds time to care about other people, it's just amazing to me. I just feel like I'm not helping her. I should be doing something more."

"Hannah, you *are* doing something for her. There's evidence of that in the fact that she cares so much about you. Maybe we give our patients the freedom to be themselves. It seems this woman has spent her life being motherly and taking care of people."

"She has!" Hannah agrees.

"And, guess what?" I continue. "Here's a lovely young woman showing up, that she can reach out to, but without a sense of obligation. I'm sure that if you were to ask her, she would be very clear about what you've meant to her in her life."

Hannah adds, "Every time I walk in she says, 'Thank you so much for taking the time to see me.' It's like she doesn't realize I'm seeing her because I genuinely care about her, not because she's a hospice patient. I keep looking for signs of an issue that she needs to deal with before she passes, but I don't see any."

"Do you envision talking with your patient about these issues so *she* can deal with it or so *you* can deal with it?"

Hannah pauses to think for a moment. "It's probably so that *I* can deal with it," she replies looking genuinely surprised. As Hannah talks herself through this realization, her voice rises with emotion. "I honestly believe that she's okay with it, but I'm not. I'm *not* okay with her leaving. I don't want her to go! I see her interact with the other patients in the home, and I just think it's unfair. I want it to be a good process for her. I think if we would talk about it, it would be better for me, because I would know she's not in anguish."

I interject. "But it occurs to me that even if she were to say, 'Hannah, it's fine. I'm ready to go and meet my God. I've had a good life. I'm 90 and I'm ready to go ....'" I trail off.

"I wouldn't believe her!" Hannah laughs, recognizing the contradiction in what she is saying and her role as a hospice volunteer. "I'm not okay with that."

"You wouldn't just suddenly turn around and say, 'Oh, okay. See ya later!'"

"Like, 'Oh, I feel better now?'" Hannah laughs ruefully. "No. I wouldn't."

"In my mind," I say, carefully. "I think that rather than asking Patrice if you're doing enough for your patient, it's more important for you to talk to Patrice about your own feelings about your patient's death."

"Yeah," Hannah agrees. "I may need to talk to Patrice about that, too, because I'm very worried about it. This is supposed to be a good experience for me and for the patient—a growing experience. I'm worried and I don't want to be, but having that conversation with her is so important that I don't want to miss anything. At the same time, if I was to walk in there this afternoon and she said, 'Hannah, I want to talk about what's going to happen when I pass,' I would probably just die! I'd be like, 'Now? Can I call Patrice first and then I'll get back to you on that?' So, I do think I'm a little confused about what our goals are and what we're supposed to help them with, if anything. I probably need clarification."

"But I'm going to put you on the spot here, Hannah. I understand what you're saying about wanting clarification, but you needed no guidelines to establish and build this relationship, including the really sweet intimacy that you have with Miss Elliott. You just followed your heart, right? And you did what came naturally."

"Yeah," Hannah sounds unconvinced.

I continue, "Then why do we feel—because I often feel the same way— why do we feel we need rules to follow as soon as that explicit conversation comes up?"

"I think for me it's the fear of saying the wrong thing," Hannah responds, "of not providing her with the comfort that she wants. I want to make her passing easier, and perhaps there is no right thing to say. It's not like you say A, and then if she responds this way, you say B, but if she responds this way, you say C."

"The flow chart?!" I laugh.

"Yes!" Hannah exclaims. "If we had that conversation the first day I went there, I probably wouldn't have thought twice about it because my heart wasn't involved yet. But now, I'm so frightened about not saying the right things for her, and what she needs is probably just—what do I truly feel? Not, what would hospice want me to say, but what do I think about it?

"But when there's something on the line," Hannah continues, "you get scared. Just like I do in the courtroom—my bar number is always on the line. I like structure. I like to establish boundaries so that I know I'm okay if I stay within the line. But with personal relationships, like when you're a hospice volunteer, there are no guidelines. There may be no right or wrong things to say, but I don't think you lose the fear. We took a training course, but I didn't feel prepared. I was thinking, 'I can't have a conversation about these things with anybody!'"

"I know. I felt the same way," I agree.

"I felt like saying, 'Come with me on my first few visits and I'll feel better!'"

"Yes! Give me a grade. How am I doing?" I laugh because I realize how similar Hannah and I are, and that it is no coincidence that she is an attorney and I am finishing my doctoral degree—both high achievers who have learned how to play by the rules. In hospice we are learning how to proceed in a context beyond rules.

My mind returns to the question at hand and I suggest, "Well, I think what you said about the impact of the relationship is really important. Think of it this way: if that conversation arose, it would be because the relationship that you've established is a safe place for your patient. It's because of who you are, not just because you're there or because you have the answers."

"That's true," Hannah agrees. "I never thought about that until you just said it. Obviously they wouldn't have that conversation with us unless they felt it was safe, and our own opinions were important. Although it's obvious, it never occurred to me until you just said it."

"I guess the only question is what if the patient doesn't need to talk about it, but you do? I think that's when we turn to hospice as our support. I think the hospice philosophy says that it's got to come from the patient. If they don't want to talk about it, there's nothing to say they *must* explicate their feelings about death to somebody before they die. And yet, people who love someone who's dying need to make sense of it, because they're the ones who'll be left behind."

"You're stuck here," Hannah adds.

I continue, "And maybe one day you'll feel some strong emotion and she'll ask you about it. Who's to say that's not the perfect thing to happen? For me, even these interviews are an example of how a conversation can be a sense-making process for the two of us. I might be doing the research, but I wouldn't have these ideas to write down without conversations with you and the others. Perhaps that can happen with hospice patients, too."

Hannah nods in agreement. "And with all that we've spoken about, as scared as I am about her passing, I'm very grateful to have had the opportunity to be with her. I wouldn't trade that, no matter what the outcome. So, I guess it's all worth it—for me anyway."

"Maybe our patients sense that this is meaningful for us, and that becomes a gift to them, too. How nice to think that even at the end we can build a connection with another person."

Hannah and I talk a little more about her call to Patrice. I note that Hannah's focus remains on learning more about how to help Miss Elliott, and my focus remains on Hannah's anticipation of grief when her patient dies. We have tackled some important questions during the course of our discussion, and I feel we have reached a level of comfort with our conclusions. Nevertheless, the questions of 'How close is too close?' and 'How do I talk to my patient about their death?' continue to run through my mind after the interview, and I feel sure the same is true for Hannah.

DOROTHY'S FIGHTING SPIRIT

We can't leave for our regular trip to the restaurant today, because Dorothy has an appointment with a respiratory therapist. This is the first time I've seen Dorothy being evaluated in this way. Terry and I both watch carefully as this new nurse administers the tests.

"Okay, Dorothy," she says, "I want you to take a deep breath in, then put this tube in your mouth and blow out until you hear a beep, like this." The nurse demonstrates.

"I'll try," Dorothy says.

As I watch Dorothy put her mouth around the large tube, I am reminded of the one time that I had a bout of asthma following a respiratory infection. The doctor made me do one of these peak flow tests, and I found it terribly difficult to blow into the machine. I felt as though I was suffocating, and the same feeling returns to me as I watch Dorothy.

"Keep going, keep going," the nurse prompts.

Dorothy suddenly inhales, and the test is not completed.

"You have to keep breathing out until the machine beeps," the nurse says.

"I'll try," Dorothy responds. "But if I can't do it, I can't do it."

The second attempt is similarly unsuccessful, then Dorothy manages to complete the third test perfectly, and the nurse records the results on a chart. Just as I feel relieved that the process is over, the nurse says, "Okay, I need two readings, so if you can do it again, just like you did it before, we'll be done."

Terry looks over at me. We can both see that the tests are making Dorothy impatient and physically exhausted.

"I thought I got it that time!" Dorothy exclaims.

"You did, Dorothy," the nurse replies, gently. "But I need two readings. I think you've got the hang of it now, so this will only take a second."

Dorothy glares at the nurse and picks up the breathing tube again.

"Okay, now, take a deep breath in, and blow, blow, blow, blow ...." The nurse coaches Dorothy like a child.

I can see that Dorothy is out of breath and she suddenly inhales again, before the beeper sounds. This is torture.

"We didn't get it," the nurse says.

"If I can't do it, I can't do it," Dorothy says. "There's no use trying again. It's impossible."

Terry, clearly distressed, says to the nurse, "Why can't you go with the reading you got the first time?"

"It's more accurate to take the average of two," the nurse tries to explain. Then she looks at Dorothy, who has folded her arms and has evidently decided not to give it another try. "I suppose we can just go with the one reading we got."

"That's good," Dorothy says. "Because I'm not doing that again. When a person has to breathe, they have to *breathe*, for Pete's sake!"

I smile to myself. So much for my feelings of protectiveness toward Dorothy! I do feel bad for the nurse, who has been very patient and kind, and is just trying to do her job. I'm also glad that Dorothy can stand up for herself. I get the impression that if Dorothy does end up in the hospital for some reason, or is faced with a situation she's not comfortable with, she will make her needs known. Her body may be frail, but her spirit is as strong as ever.

SHYANNE

As I drive to Shyanne's neighborhood, I listen to her interview on the cassette player for the third time. The sound of our voices fills my car as I work my way through the morning traffic to the south side of town. I am struck by Shyanne's ability to share evocative stories ripe with metaphor and insight. This ability seems more than the residue of her profession as a counselor, and more like a spiritual gift. We meet at the same coffee shop as before. I step inside from the bright sunlight, and as soon as my eyes adjust to the shade, I see Shyanne. We greet each other with smiles and hugs, then settle in.

"Well," Shyanne begins, "my patient died on the very last day in July. After the first interview, we spent a lot of time learning from each other, and teaching each other. A couple of months ago, she fell and broke her leg, which then failed to heal, and she was put into an ALF, an assisted living facility. It was a source of pride for her that she lived on her own, and her attitude was that the cancer was not going to get the better of her. Once she got to the ALF, she gave up, and that's when the struggle began for me. Originally, I resisted volunteering in a nursing home, and suddenly, there I was." Shyanne throws up her hands in a classic gesture of surrender.

In our first interview, Shyanne spoke eloquently about what it had meant to her, a white, former South African, to visit an elderly African American woman in one of the poorest areas of town. I sense that she considers her patient's move to an ALF as a similarly portentous event—one that brought a challenge and an opportunity for growth.

Shyanne continues, "For a long time we tried to get her healed and transferred back to her apartment. Then, I realized it had to be about her and not me, and she needed to be at the ALF for a while. I was not impressed with the care that she got. She was in a lot of pain for a long time until we got in and said, 'It's not working.' She became quiet and not really herself. Food was always a big thing for her; it was an occasion, but she stopped finding pleasure in the things she usually did. She lost a lot of her faculties; she would tell me in expletives to get out of her room because she didn't know me. It was pretty interesting for me, but I realized it was part of the disease process. The cancer had gone into her brain and into her bones.

"We had tried to get someone, family, anyone, to come, but at the time I was the only person going to see her, and no one appeared. She originally said that she had no family, but we found out she did have a daughter on the streets and a distant cousin. It was hard for me to understand how a daughter could completely abandon her mother like that.

"I had just seen her a few days earlier when I got the call. They told me she was close to death, and if I was going to come, I had to come right away. I drove up and I was there when she died. A couple of days later, these relatives climbed out of the woodwork to see if there was any money left." Shyanne's slender fingers creep lightly across the tabletop in a gesture that communicates exactly how she pictures these relatives. "That's what they wanted. I had to distance myself and focus on the fact that I was there and she was not alone when she died, which was her biggest fear. She died peacefully; I think she decided that it was time. The staff was wonderful. One nurse in particular was there, rubbing her hands and saying it was okay to let go, and there was a peaceful place waiting for her. She took one more breath and—exited. Hospice has called me a couple of times but, because the last few months were so agonizing, her death was almost a relief."

"So, how long did you spend with her when she was dying? Was it hours?"

Shyanne shakes her head. "Fifteen minutes. They called and I was in the middle of dinner. I got up and left, was there, and she stopped breathing."

"Really?" I'm very surprised. During our training we learned that vigil volunteers are scheduled on 3-hour shifts, sometimes for a day or two, when a patient is actively dying. I also remember a colleague, Ginny Conley (2001), presenting a paper that discussed the phenomenon where people who are dying seem to make conscious choices regarding the timing of their death, even when they have been unconscious for days or months.

"Maybe she knew that you were there?" I wonder aloud.

"I have no way of knowing," Shyanne replies. "But the most ironic thing happened. My patient had just died, and I was feeling sad about all the things she never got to experience, thinking, 'Is this all there is to this 70-year-old woman? What evidence do we have that she was ever here? What imprint has she made?' I was getting really heavy and really angry. Then, on the other side of the curtain was a little old lady asking for Jello and ice cream. She knew what was happening, but life goes on. The nurse went in to ask what kind of ice cream she wanted, and it gave me this little wake-up call, that life does go on. Clarice may be dead, but the patient next door is still concerned about what flavor of ice cream she's going to get!"

"It's pretty amazing," I reflect. "During the last interview, you talked about your fear of death, and now you've faced it! You had a close relationship, went into it completely and open-heartedly, and now you're on the other side, and it's okay. There are other people I've interviewed whose patients have died, but you're the only one who's actually been there."

Shyanne nods silently.

I pause a moment, then say, "I still have my first patient."

"Oh, wow!" Shyanne responds.

"I'm feeling a little anxious about what's going to happen."

"How is the disease progressing?" Shyanne asks.

"Very slowly. But once or twice she's had these spells. She lost her ability to express herself for an hour or so. I couldn't understand her at all, and it scared me a lot. I've talked to her nurse and she said, 'Dorothy is in complete denial about the disease. You have to be prepared.' And I don't think I am prepared!"

This incident has been on my mind since it happened. Jackie's warning only made me feel more worried.

Shyanne replies, "I don't think you can ever be prepared. Death doesn't ask permission; it's there when it's there. One of the advantages of getting close to a patient is that you can at least open the door to communication about death. At first, Clarice wouldn't talk about it."

"And then what happened?" I ask, attentively.

"I *needed* to talk about it," Shyanne declares. "So, I started to bring things up and eventually she was deteriorating to the point where the social worker at the ALF needed to know what kinds of measures she wanted—tube feeding, CPR—and she would not talk about it for weeks. Eventually, I asked her directly. She would change the subject, but I kept at it, being specific. 'If your heart stops, do you want them to start your heart again?' She would ramble about when she was a child and getting prickles in her feet. Then I would bring her back again. I had the paper and I said, 'They need to know.'"

"So, they asked you to pursue that with her?"

"They were not getting anywhere with her," Shyanne shakes her head. "She just wouldn't communicate with them, or she would give them the runaround, or they were not tenacious, or didn't have time. We got to where she couldn't make medical decisions and the social worker solicited for me to become her health care surrogate. That was a lot for me. I had to go and think about it, because I really didn't want to get that involved."

I am surprised that she was put in that position. "What did hospice say about it?"

"Hospice wasn't involved when that happened. Because she had fallen, she needed full-time nursing. Until she reached a certain point, she got that through Medicaid. After she recovered sufficiently, or declined, hospice could take over."

I know that hospice strongly discourages volunteer visits once patients leave hospice, so I was curious. "You continued to visit her?"

"Occasionally, yes. And I would see things that bothered me that needed to be taken care of, like pain medication. She wasn't getting a high enough dose and someone had to say, 'It's *not normal* for her to be lying there in a fetal position. It's *not normal* for her to have her body so strung out waiting for her next dose. I don't care if the doctor says it's a strong dose, it's not strong enough for her.' So, after I thought about it, I went back and signed some papers. In the end, Clarice got pain control and they weren't forcing her to eat any more. She was in a place where she was ready to go.

"Her move to the ALF made it a little messy, because when her disease had progressed to a certain level, they called hospice to say her Medicaid was running out and to ask, 'Can you step in?' So, hospice evaluated her and came back in; then, after a few days in hospice, she died. It was just a really weird, convoluted situation I never thought I'd get involved in, but what it boiled down to is that she had no one else. I spent 6 months getting to know her, and no one else was going to be there for her in that way."

"So, how did you feel about being put in that position? I know as volunteers we put ourselves there, but you took on a more extreme level of responsibility."

Shyanne nods as she replies. "That's an issue that I brought up with the staff at the ALF. I said, 'I'm just the volunteer here. I'm going home to my perfect little family and leaving you with the mess, because a few hours a week is all I can give you.' But then I thought, 'Someone has to take a stand and say, "I'll do it."' We're all so afraid of getting involved—even volunteers. You give this amount of your time and then you withdraw, which you must, but I'm so tired of people not taking a stand. I think we're all supposed to help others, to give happiness, to give love, and Clarice had no one but strangers doing that for her. It was also important for me to be involved with someone who was going to die, and all the pain that involved, and also for Clarice, so that she knew she had someone on her side."

I want to know more about how Shyanne and Clarice interacted, particularly once Clarice started to decline and "lose her faculties," as Shyanne put it. "What were the visits like?"

I catch a wistful look as Shyanne considers my question. "I read books to her. I read the Bible. That was interesting to me because I'm a New Testament person and she loved the Old Testament. Especially the book where everybody begets everybody else—she loved that stuff! She liked to be touched, because she said they only touch her when they need to give her medication. So, she liked to have her hair brushed or her arms or legs rubbed, and just talking. She loved to hear about my kids. I told her once that I have a flower garden and every time I saw her after that, without fail, we talked about my garden. It was a connection for us, a bridge. Over and over she'd have me describe the flowers. What colors? Did they like shade? All to a level of detail that I didn't even have for her. I would bring her flowers from the garden, and that would perk her up, but eventually there was no reaction from her."

Shyanne smiles, "I used to smuggle apple pie in from McDonald's, those crispy fried things? She just loved them. She would gobble them up, but she wouldn't eat the healthy food that they gave her. She wanted fried chicken and apple pie. What's it going to do, kill her?" Shyanne shakes her head at the occasional insanity in the medical mindset.

I concur, wholeheartedly. "I have a colleague, Ginny Conley, who wrote a paper called, 'Eat the Ice Cream First.'"

"Oh!" Shyanne sighs sympathetically as she hears the title.

I continue, "It's about the end of life. She argues, when somebody is that ill, let them have their dessert, or their Jack Daniels, if that's what they want!"

"Who cares?!" Shyanne chimes in. "I'm not going to try to stick the Boost down her, or whatever energy drink they give her. If she wants fried chicken, let's give her Kentucky Fried Chicken. She eats two mouthfuls and she's happy."

Shyanne pauses a moment, then continues. "I understand the staff's position. They have to really dwell in their head to get their job done, to remain detached, to maintain that level of professionalism. They don't remain in their heart too much, but that's so they survive."

"And what did you bring that was a contrast to that?" I prompt.

"To me, Clarice was not just a number or a chart or a 'to do' list; she was a person. When I went to her, I didn't just go to give something; I went there to get something, and it was a mutual exchange of conversation, of energy, of laughter. And she gave me little pearls along the way that I'll never *ever* be without. I also think it was safe for her to be really honest with me about the pain, or her fear, or ask whether that stuff in the Bible really was true. I was someone to talk to, and 99% of the time, I had no answers. I just had to sit there and nod my head and say, 'I know, I know,' because I really had no answers."

"What do you think was the most challenging moment for you?"

"There were many moments of challenge," Shyanne replies. "I think more than anything it was the bureaucracy, the red tape, the paperwork, and the insurance. 'We can't pay for it every 2 hours, we can only pay for it every 4 hours,' regardless of whether she's writhing in agony—which just makes no sense to me. In my mind, she did not get to die a good death."

"Really?" I'm very surprised.

"No," Shyanne responds emphatically. "Because she was in pain up to just a few days before she died because of people not wanting to change medication orders, because they felt she was getting enough. So what if she got too much? What is the worst thing that can happen? That she could sleep for the next 4 days? It made no sense to me why someone should be in so much agony that she couldn't keep any of her food down, or control any of her body processes, and go through bouts of shivering or being boiling hot.

"Like I said before, the true agony was in the time preceding her death, and when she died, she looked so peaceful. She was smiling, free of all of this. There was an interesting expression on her face; she looked—done. It was the first time in 4 months that I'd seen her face relaxed, because it was always tensed waiting for the next wave of pain. I finally got to see her as she really is, but I had to wait until death to see it."

I consider the goals of hospice for a moment, and then ask, "Was there something that you contributed that helped bring her closer to 'the good death'?"

Shyanne responds, "I think I did because she did not die alone. She was afraid that she'd die as a number in some bed with strangers all around her, and no one would know she was dead. She thought that they'd come the next morning and realize that she had died. I didn't really do anything. I hadn't been in the room with someone who was dying before, and I didn't know what to do. All I knew to do was to be myself and give myself, to rub her hand or her forehead. The nurse had some really interesting advice about what to say to her. Clarice got to the point where she was breathing eight times per minute and the nurse knew; she said it would be any time."

"What advice did she give you that was interesting?" I probe.

"She said, 'Just think what a good time this is for her. She's finally able to go. It's okay to be sad, but realize that sadness is for you. When we cry, it's because we're left alone without that person.' If she had been laughing, and talking, no pain, and eating apple pie the day before she died, then it would have been very sad; instead, there was a sense of relief."

Something still nags at me regarding what Clarice's nurse had said. I share my thoughts with Shyanne. "You were able to be relieved for her, but if this was my father or my mother, I don't think I could think as that nurse did. You know? 'Don't be sad, be glad for them, because you're just being sad for yourself.' I think I'd be saying, 'Of course I'm sad for myself!'"

Shyanne grins. "Stupid woman!" she chimes in.

"Yeah!" I continue. "How can you tell me not to be sad?"

Shyanne smiles and nods, then clarifies. "I don't think you're supposed to be that detached for family. That's the definition of family, for me: to truly care and want someone around all the time. You have an emotional investment in family; they enrich your life and you see how they enrich the world. I never got to see how Clarice interacted with the world. I just saw a very small view of her with me. I never got to see who she really was in her life. She was always in her disease when I knew her, and I knew that they were two very different people."

I agree. "My patient's enriched my life, too, although it's hard for me to articulate exactly how. I went on vacation a couple of weeks ago and when I got back, I called her and she said, 'Well, I missed you, honey.' And I thought, 'Wow.' I was looking forward to our visit, and she missed me. From being total strangers, it's pretty amazing how far we've come in 6 months."

I ask, "To what extent did you have that dying process in your mind when you interacted with her. You said you talked about the flowers and I remember the beautiful story you told about cooking squash ...."

Shyanne laughs.

"... and finding those moments of connection," I continue. "I've been surprised by how little I've thought about death with my patient."

Shyanne agrees. "In the foremost of my mind was touching her and enriching her in some way during each visit—giving her something she may not have had before, being instrumental in her smiling more that day, or being relatively pain free, or feeling better about herself. I really didn't think about the disease; it became a distant relative in the background, and she, as a person, was why I was there."

"I like that image of the distant relative in the background," I reflect. "It's as if you accept that as part of the context, and you don't even have to worry about it any more." It occurs to me later that this image is an interesting contrast to the proverbial "elephant in the corner"—the thing that is huge but we pretend that it isn't there and refuse to talk about it. I wonder how Shyanne and I were making the distinction between the "distant relative" meaning that we focused on the patient, and the "elephant in the corner," which meant denial of the disease.

Shyanne continues, "You have to do your best to separate the disease from the person, because if you allow the disease to completely take over, you start becoming angry and asking questions: 'I don't understand why this is happening. This isn't fair.' Most of the time, I managed to focus on the person that I knew. She still had beautiful hands, and she still had a great laugh when she was laughing. Or that twinkle in her eye when she did have her eyes open. I was able to focus on the good things. Sometimes I went into that dark, scary place where I was angry at the disease. I got angry with her for not taking care of her body; if she hadn't eaten all that junk and smoked and blah, blah, blah. Those were little lapses into my insanity, then I was able to come back and say, 'She's smiling today. And that's great.' And I didn't think of the cancer."

I observe, "When you're close to somebody, in some ways the disease does become overwhelming. You see the disparity between the person you've had a relationship with and what's happening with the disease. It starts to obliterate the person. I think that's what's meant by 'holistic care' as a contrast with the biomedical model, which is all about the disease. We can have a relationship with the disease, but it's not really going to help anybody."

"We don't honor that person," Shyanne adds. "They are a human being, they've walked on the earth, they've touched people, they've breathed the air, they've had children, they've had relationships, they've created things, and that's what we need to connect with."

We are running short of time, and this is a wonderful observation to conclude our discussion. I say, "Shyanne, you are an amazing person to interview!"

Shyanne laughs, "Good! I'm glad. That's great, Elissa."

We talk a little more as we pack up and prepare to leave. Shyanne is taking some time off from volunteering while she travels. We discuss the possibility of a third interview, and then say our goodbyes.

BACK ON OXYGEN

After missing one of our weekly visits because of a conference in Atlanta, I am surprised to see Dorothy back on oxygen when I return.

"Hi Dorothy!" I exclaim as I come through the door.

"Well, hello there!" Dorothy says as she stands up from her chair. She walks over to me and we hug. "I missed you, honey!" she says.

"I missed you, too, Dorothy," I respond.

We sit and talk for a little while as *Texas Justice* plays on the television. Then I comment, "I see you're back on the oxygen."

Dorothy rolls her eyes, "Yes, they said I should use it more, so Terry makes me keep it on, now. But I really don't see that it makes any difference. I just keep it on to make her happy."

I nod in agreement, but I don't say anything more. I wish I knew more about the medical decisions that are being made regarding Dorothy's condition. I don't know how to interpret this change. Does it mean that she is getting worse again?

When it is time for lunch, Dorothy takes off her oxygen and heads for the door.

"Shouldn't we take this with us?" I ask, picking up Dorothy's portable oxygen tank.

"No, I don't need it," Dorothy says, continuing on her journey out to the car.

I hesitate for a moment trying to decide between two undesirable options: I can defy Dorothy and what she wants to do, or I can risk facing a situation where we need her oxygen and don't have it. I think about the hospice principle of responding to what the patient wants, and set the oxygen tank back down beside the sofa. I also decide that the next time we go out, I will tell Dorothy that *I* would feel more comfortable if we had the oxygen with us in the car.

Our lunch proceeds as usual, without incident. When we return home, we sit outside in the breezeway and Dorothy will not put her oxygen back on. However, as soon as she sees Terry's car coming around the corner, she suggests that we go inside and is wearing her oxygen again by the time Terry opens the door.

It occurs to me that if I were Terry, I might find these antics very frustrating. As it is, though, I perceive Dorothy's refusal to wear her oxygen as an indication that she is fighting to live life on her own terms. I have to admire and appreciate her determination.

THE DOLLAR STORE

At the Crossroads Diner today, Dorothy and I share stories about our respective Thanksgiving holidays. Terry has been picking up some extra work and has been very busy, so a week ago, I was a little concerned that they had made no plans. Today, I discover from Dorothy that they ended up with two turkeys— one from LifePath and one from the organization that delivers lunches to Dorothy. At the last minute, both of Terry's daughters—Leslie and Sharon—decided to come into town to share Thanksgiving with Terry and Dorothy. Unfortunately, Len was on the road, but it sounds like the women had a wonderful time together.

On our way home from the diner, Dorothy asks if we can stop at the dollar store so she can buy some hand lotion. She tells me that she and Stan used to shop at this store all the time. We make a careful selection of the best deal on lotion, comparing ingredients and sizes. We look at a few items as we make our way to the counter, and then Dorothy makes her purchase.

I think about how this simple event of buying lotion seemed to lift Dorothy's spirits, and my own. I think about how little control Dorothy really has over her life, and I see how happy it makes her to be able to visit a store and choose her own hand lotion. For the next several days, I try to pay attention to all the freedoms and opportunities I have that I take for granted—and I declare it my own private week of giving thanks. I even try to appreciate being stuck in traffic, because it means that I have somewhere I want to be and a car to get me there. I think about how simple it was to give Dorothy something that made her happy—we didn't have to go to Disney World, or spend vast amounts of money, or a great deal of time. All it took was 20 minutes and a trip to the dollar store. Given my initial concerns about doing something to brighten Dorothy's day, I am surprised to realize that it can be this easy, and that it has probably been this easy from the very beginning.

REFLECTIONS: DIALECTICS AND FINDING BALANCE IN THE VOLUNTEER ROLE

The stories in this chapter illustrate some of the dilemmas faced by hospice volunteers as they strive to establish relationships with their patients that will be positive for both parties. So far, I have only briefly indicated some of the inherent contradictions or *dialectic tensions* within hospice, and specifically within the relationships between hospice volunteers and patients. In this reflection, I will define dialectics for readers who are unfamiliar with the concept, and describe how dialectics can help to explain the volunteers' experience of needing to find balance while being drawn in different directions simultaneously. I conclude the chapter by highlighting similarities between the dialectics of friendship (Rawlins, 1992) and the dialectic tensions encountered by the volunteers.

Rather than constituting a theory in and of itself, dialectics can be more accurately conceived as a metatheoretical orientation that guides a range of theories across several disciplines including philosophy, political science, organizational studies, sociology, as well as the study of personal relationships (Baxter & Montgomery, 1996). What dialectical theories have in common is that they emphasize the unity of opposing tendencies within the domain of human activity. In relationship studies, these opposing forces center on the relationship between self and other—for example, the desire to be autonomous and the desire for connection, the desire for both novelty and predictability in a relationship, or the desire to express one's thoughts and feelings and also to keep them private. Rather than suggesting that there is one "resolution" to these opposing tensions, or even that these forces exist as static sets of matched binary opposites, the relational dialectics perspective argues that relationships are affected by overlapping forces of coming together (centripetal) and coming apart (centrifugal) (Baxter & Montgomery, 1996, p. 44). Thus, relational dialectics emphasizes complexity, dynamic movement, and change in ways that other theoretical perspectives do not. It also provides a language and a framework for discussing and clarifying aspects of relationships that can be confusing, contradictory, and often hard to come to terms with—as illustrated by the stories in this chapter.

Hannah's primary concern in this second interview was with the impact of her growing attachment to her patient, Miss Elliott. At first,

Hannah focused on the question of whether she was doing anything to help her patient "come to terms" with dying, and also whether she was receiving more benefit from the relationship than Miss Elliott. As we probed a little deeper through the interview, Hannah also revealed her growing anxiety about losing her relationship with Miss Elliott when she died. Hannah was caught in two dialectics; first, she questioned the balance of giving and receiving in the relationship, and second, she was concerned that her attachment (holding on) to Miss Elliott would stand in the way of her goal as a hospice volunteer, which involved support- ing Miss Elliott as she died (letting go). These two dilemmas overlapped because the more Hannah "received" from the relationship, the less she felt capable of letting go of the relationship.

Hannah described her relationship with Miss Elliott as "more than" a volunteer–patient relationship; in fact, Hannah's descriptions and the dilemmas she faced stem from the emerging friendship that she and Miss Elliot shared. Rawlins (1992) proposes that ideal-typical friend- ships in our culture are distinguished from other kinds of close relation- ships by a number of characteristics, including equality, voluntary and mutual involvement, and affective ties. Because of the emphasis of our hospice training, Hannah entered her relationship with Miss Elliott with the goal of *helping* her or *giving* to her—not the other way around. As their affection for one another grew and they became mutually in- volved in each others' lives, the relationship took on friendship dimen- sions of equality rather than the helping relationship that Hannah initially envisioned. As a quality of friendship, equality is affected by the dialectic of instrumentality and affection (Rawlins, 1992), wherein it becomes impossible to make sharp distinctions between selfish and selfless acts, and between acts of affection and acts of assistance. As I suggested to Hannah, for a person like Miss Elliott who had spent her life helping others, Hannah's willingness to receive Miss Elliott's care and affection may have been the greatest gift that Hannah could give her.

What complicated the matter for Hannah was her own reluctance to surrender the idea that she should be enacting her role according to a hospice ideal— that she did not have the resources to respond in the right way, particularly in relation to talking to Miss Elliott about her death. Hannah was willing to engage this conversation only in the con- text of helping Miss Elliott, but not if the conversation was for Hannah's comfort and peace of mind. What would have been a natural—albeit emotionally challenging—conversation emerging in a conventional friendship became difficult to negotiate within the hospice guidelines of acting *only* in the interests of the patient. Although this principle makes sense in the hypothetical, and is, I believe, crucial in the early stages of a relationship between a volunteer and a patient, in cases like

Hannah's where a mutual, equal, and reciprocal friendship emerges it seems unnecessarily limiting to insist on maintaining an unequal helping stance.

Perhaps because the circumstances were quite different, and because she was no longer within the province of hospice regulations, Shyanne's responses to Clarice's needs were very different. What stands out in my mind was Shyanne's answer to my question about how she talked to Clarice about dying. Shyanne said, "I *needed* to talk about it." Rather than wondering what was appropriate according to hospice guidelines, Shyanne recognized that in order to take care of Clarice as she died, she needed to address the issue explicitly with her. Although she risked alienating Clarice and upsetting the relationship that they had established, Shyanne's stories suggest that they had developed a degree of trust, which allowed Shyanne to feel confident about engaging a topic Clarice wanted to avoid. The dialectic of expressiveness and protectiveness in friendship (Rawlins, 1992) describes the delicate dance of managing appropriate levels of candor in order to preserve the dignity of each person and the quality of the relationship. My own response to this dilemma in my relationship with Dorothy was very different. I did not question Dorothy about her use of oxygen or anything else about her disease. For better or worse, part of our friendship relied on my compliance in *not* focusing on Dorothy's physical condition, which in turn meant not asking about it. Although our culture tends to value unremitting openness in close relationships, at least in the ideal, there is no doubt that a certain degree of restraint or protectiveness can also contribute to positive outcomes in a close relationship (Bochner, 1995).

Shyanne's story also illustrates tensions that can arise between hospice organizational regulations and a volunteer's sense of justice, commitment, and responsibility. While Clarice's rehabilitation was handled by the ALF, she was temporarily transferred out of the hospice program, and according to hospice guidelines, Shyanne's relationship with Clarice should not have continued. However, Shyanne recognized that Clarice needed someone, regardless of the change in her status. Shyanne became Clarice's only advocate in the ALF; she fought to ensure that Clarice received adequate care, particularly in relation to pain control, and was present when Clarice died. Hospice-as-organization would no doubt disagree with Shyanne's decision to become so involved in Clarice's care; although many individuals who work for hospice would no doubt understand entirely why she chose to take on so much responsibility. To the extent that Shyanne and Clarice had built a friendship that existed outside the obligations of hospice volunteering that brought them together initially, that friendship extended beyond the boundaries of hospice services. As Shyanne said, "What it boiled down to is that she had no one else. I had spent 6 months getting to know her and no one else was going to be there for her in that way."

The last point I would like to make about friendship in relation to hospice volunteers and patients is that although many of the participants in this study (and their patients) used the word *friend* to describe their relationship, the formal dimensions of the volunteer role limits its appropriateness as a descriptor. Specifically, as Rawlins (1992) points out, "friendship can not be imposed on people; it is an ongoing human association voluntarily developed and privately negotiated" (p. 9). Both the volunteers and the hospice patients volunteer to enter the relationship, and both have a choice about whether or not they want to accept a given arrangement, but the boundaries of that relationship are (or are intended to be) prescribed by hospice. For example, volunteers were advised to maintain certain formalities like calling before visits, visiting for less than 4 hours per week, and submitting notes to account for each contact with our patients. Within such boundaries, whether or not a friendship emerges is privately negotiated, and must be sanctioned by both the volunteer and patient. When Dorothy introduced me as "her friend" to Debbie, the server at the diner, I recognized it as a privilege given to me by Dorothy as a result of the time we had spent together up to that point. In that moment of naming me her friend, the meaning of our interaction shifted so that the activities of volunteering—meeting weekly, talking, sitting together, going out—took on the voluntary qualities of friendship, while the formal dimensions of hospice volunteering became less significant. Although Dorothy did not initially choose me to be her friend, at some point she chose to invite me into the circle of her life as a friend, which is something that cannot be expected or imposed. The idea of finding balance within a dialectic does not imply finding an ideal point somewhere in between the two extremes—for example, an imaginary point at which one is neither holding on nor letting go. Just as tightrope walkers and dancers find balance through movement and constant engagement with one another, finding balance in a relationship is a dynamic and reflexive process of responding to the demands of the context, our needs, and those of the other person, with a sense of the past, present, and future relationship. As such, finding balance implies improvisation wherein we are fully present and ready to respond in the moment, recognizing that at any given time we may be influenced by opposing or contradictory inclinations. As I learned from my acting classes, improvisation requires us to resist becoming stuck in the dilemma of choices; rather, we must keep going, always in the affirmative. The answer is always yes.

PART IV

Communication at the Time of Death

In Part IV, I present stories from the last set of interviews I conducted with the volunteers in my study and from the end of my relationship with Dorothy. In these chapters, I aim to bring a sense of meaning and closure to the stories. In the final chapter, I draw conclusions about communication at the end of life by connecting the narratives to relevant communication and sociological theory.

In three episodes, chapter 9 recounts the last visits I spent with Dorothy and her family, as well as the personal ritual I enacted as my private farewell to Dorothy. Chapter 10 weaves together observations from the volunteers who participated in my study. This chapter provides an update for each volunteer's story, presents the volunteers' thoughts on the meaning of their experiences, and foreshadows the academic reflections in the subsequent chapter. Chapter 11 focuses on two aspects of the study. In the first section, I present my interpretation of the volunteers' journey through the first year, specifically as it relates to our attitudes toward hospice and hospice volunteering. In the second section, I return to the original question that prompted the research: How do we communicate with people who are at the end of life? And, I pose the closely related question regarding the nature of the volunteers' contributions to end-of-life care in hospice. The answers to both questions are linked by the concept of *social dying* as an experience that can accompany approaching death for those who are dying, and which we can alleviate through communication that is grounded in the principle of *being there* for those who are at the end of life.

9

Endings

SLOWING DOWN

When I return from Christmas vacation in January, things continue in much the same way that they always have, except that Dorothy is using her oxygen all the time. Just after I have been visiting Dorothy for a year, something changes.

I arrive at Dorothy's place and Terry lets me into the apartment. Terry tells me immediately that Dorothy is up and dressed, looking forward to going out to the restaurant, but she has fallen asleep in her chair.

"I should wake her up," Terry says. "She'll want to see you."

Alarmed by the change in Dorothy's routine, I also notice that she seems quite breathless as she sleeps.

"Mom," Terry says, gently but loud enough for Dorothy to hear. "Mom, Elissa's here."

Dorothy blinks several times as she opens her eyes, and asks, "Who is it?"

"Your babysitter's here," Terry says, a little louder.

Once I see that she recognizes me, I walk over to give Dorothy a hug. "Hi, Dorothy. How are you doing?"

"I'm fine," Dorothy says. "How are you doing?"

"Great," I reply. "Working hard, as always, but I'm happy."

"That's good," Dorothy says. "Hope those kids aren't giving you too much trouble." She appears to lapse into a little daze as she watches the television. Although we have enacted our ritual as always, I get the feeling that Dorothy is in a different world—she's not quite here.

Terry sits watching us together, and then says: "Can you see it?"

I nod in confirmation. I assume that Terry is referring to the change in Dorothy's demeanor, but I don't feel comfortable talking about Dorothy as if she is not there, so I don't say anything else.

Terry and I talk for a little while, catching up with what's been going on in the family. Every so often, I try to engage Dorothy in conversation. She responds, but very briefly.

Then, after about 40 minutes, Dorothy says to me, "So, do you want to go get a bite to eat?"

I smile, "Yes, absolutely." I'm surprised that she wants to go, and I'm also thrilled that she feels up for it.

"Let's all go together," Terry says, pointedly. Terry accompanied Dorothy and me to lunch once before, but that was many months ago, and this time, I sense her reasons for coming to the diner stem from concern for her mother's health rather than a desire to socialize.

This time, there is no question about the oxygen. Not only does Dorothy use her oxygen during the entire trip, it is also necessary for me to drop Terry and Dorothy close to the door of the restaurant so that Dorothy does not have to walk too far. Dorothy has always been tiny, but she looks even more fragile today, her feet barely lifting from the ground to propel her forward. I watch as Terry carries the oxygen tank in one hand and gently guides her mother with her other arm curled protectively around Dorothy's shoulders.

On the surface, lunch seems the same as it always is, but I can feel that something is wrong. Dorothy seems barely aware of our presence, and when I look down at her plate, her omelet and hash browns are hardly touched.

At one point, Terry gets up to use the rest room, and I say, "Dorothy, you seem very quiet today. Is there anything on your mind that's worrying you?"

Dorothy looks at me and considers the question for a moment, then replies, "No, there's nothing on my mind that I'm worried about."

"Okay," I reply, and put my hand on hers briefly. "Just wanted to make sure everything was all right with you."

When we return home, Dorothy needs help getting to the bathroom. I sit waiting in my usual spot in the living room, and when Terry comes back, I say, "Dorothy seems terribly quiet today."

"Yes, I think she's beginning to leave us," Terry replies. "The hospice social worker came around a couple of days ago and left some brochures about what we can expect in the next few weeks."

I am surprised by how calm she sounds. I try to respond in the way that I think experienced volunteers should respond. I try to appear as though I understand what is happening to Dorothy. Inside, I feel a wave of panic flood my chest as I realize that I am not ready for her to "leave."

Dorothy calls from the bathroom, and Terry helps her to walk back to the living room, her breathing labored and movements shaky. Once settled, Dorothy sits back in her chair, closes her eyes, and leans her head back. I don't know what to say to her, and it's time for me to go.

"Dorothy," I say gently as I stand up. "I have to get back to work now." I lean over her chair and give her a hug. It's difficult for me to keep my composure as I think about what these changes mean, but I force myself to stay calm, and smile as I look into her blue-green eyes.

"Oh, okay," Dorothy says. As I reach the door, I hear her say from her chair in the corner, "I enjoyed it, honey. I always do, you know."

"Me, too, Dorothy," I reply. "I'll call in a few days."

As I pull away in my car, I surrender to the impulse to cry. I tell myself it's okay to cry, now that I'm in the privacy of my car. I wonder if this was our last lunch at the restaurant. I wonder how much time we have left. I wonder if I will see Dorothy again.

OUR LAST VISIT

I have been up since early morning, trying to be productive before I leave my apartment for a series of appointments in an unusually busy day. I sit restlessly at the computer, typing and periodically glancing at the clock in my kitchen. Slowly, the minute hand creeps toward 10 o'clock, the hour that I have planned to call Dorothy and arrange my weekly visit. I have stayed in more regular contact with Terry over the last couple of weeks, trying to stay in touch with the changes in Dorothy. I've learned that her condition is unpredictable. One day last week she was barely able to speak, so I left early and came back 2 days later. At that visit, Dorothy was as feisty as ever, still struggling, but certainly more like her self.

I look at the clock again. I remember that my first visit to Dorothy was at this hour of the morning, and then our appointments got later as I adjusted to the rhythm of her life. Visiting Dorothy has become a part of my life now.

At 10:02 a.m., I call.

"Hello?" Terry answers.

"Good morning, Terry, it's Elissa," I say. "I was just calling to make sure it was okay for me to come over to visit Dorothy."

"Ah ..." Terry hesitates.

Immediately, my stomach tightens. Dorothy's condition must be worse.

"I'm actually still trying to get her out of bed," Terry explains. "She doesn't seem to want to get up this morning."

"Would it be better for me to wait a while before I come over?" I ask.

"Yeah, that would probably be better," Terry seems relieved.

"I could wait about 45 minutes, then drive over?" I suggest.

"That'd probably be fine. Why don't you do that?" Terry says.

"Okay," I agree. "I'll be around just before 11."

"See you then," Terry hangs up the phone.

Now, I'm worried about timing. I have another commitment in the early afternoon. I had planned to arrive at Dorothy's earlier today so that I could spend 2 hours with her before leaving at noon. I don't want to cut my visit short, particularly if Dorothy is getting worse. I make myself relax and acknowledge that I can only plan my day once I find out how Dorothy is doing. If I need to adjust my plans, I can and will.

Time has been slow all morning, but it seems to go by even slower as I wait the 45 minutes before heading over to Dorothy's. As I lock my front door, I wonder if I should have called a second time to make sure it was okay. I didn't give Terry the opportunity to ask me to wait again, perhaps because I fear having to forego my visit altogether.

I am surprised when Len answers the door. I had forgotten that he was going to be at home this weekend, and he would usually be out on another job by mid-week anyway. I wonder if he's here because Dorothy has been getting worse. He smiles warmly and ushers me into the living room. I immediately notice that Dorothy is not sitting in her chair. I watch Terry out of my peripheral vision as I chat with Len about how he's been doing and how his last road trip was. Terry is busy making breakfast and laying out Dorothy's pills in the kitchen. She has not yet greeted me, nor has she acknowledged my arrival. I sense tension in the apartment, but I don't know whether it's because of Len, or me, or because of something happening with Dorothy.

"Hi Terry, how are you doing?" I ask, pointedly.

"I'm doing fine," Terry replies, glancing up briefly. "As you can see, I haven't managed to get her out of bed yet, so I don't know what kind of a visit you're going to have." Terry walks toward me wiping her hands on a towel and I try to read her face. Is she upset, frustrated, tired, scared, or a combination of all these emotions?

"I'm happy to just go back to the bedroom and sit with her for a little while if that's okay with you," I say.

Terry appears to relax a little. "Sure," she says. "That's fine with me. She's kind of out of it, but you can go ahead if you want to."

"I'd really like to," I say. It occurs to me that, as difficult as it is for me to be here, it is difficult for Terry, too. No doubt Terry was pleased to have me interact socially with Dorothy and enjoy her company, but now I will see Dorothy at her most vulnerable, no longer her feisty self. I wonder how I would feel leading someone back to see my mother confined to a bed. I hope Terry knows how much I care about both of them and that she can trust me.

Terry leads the way into Dorothy's bedroom. A couple of weeks ago, Terry described the changes she and Len had made to make it easier for Dorothy to get to her bathroom. Even so, I am surprised when I peek around Terry's shoulder and see the hospital bed at an odd angle across the room, with the foot of the bed near the door, and Dorothy lying so still.

"Mom," Terry says loudly. "Mom, you have a visitor!"

I watch Dorothy struggle to open her eyes in response to Terry. "No! I don't want them!" Her words are slurred and muffled, but her intention is very clear.

For a second, I feel the stab of disappointment because Dorothy doesn't want to see me. Then Terry says, "Wait 'til you see who it is! It's Elissa. She's come to visit with you."

I see Dorothy's eyes focus on me unsteadily, and she relaxes. For a second, I question whether this means that she is glad to see me, or if she is simply being polite. Then I realize that Dorothy, even in this condition, would not hesitate let us know if she wanted to be alone.

I move toward her, and Terry says, "You can sit right there on the bed."

"Thank you," I say to Terry as she slips out the door. "Hi Dorothy, I'm very glad to see you. You're having a rough day today, but I hope it will be okay if I just sit with you for a little while." It is more of a statement than a question, but I feel I've left enough of an opening for Dorothy to send me away if she wants to.

Dorothy tilts her had back a little on the pillow, then closes her eyes. Despite the audible flow of oxygen coming through her nose tube, I notice that Dorothy's mouth is wide open and her lungs are pulling in regular, if shallow, breaths of air. I am glad that I hear no obstruction in her breathing, but she seems to be working hard.

I slip my hand underneath hers as they taught us to do in the hospice training. Because my hand is underneath hers, Dorothy will be able to move her hand away from mine more easily if she feels uncomfortable. Her hand remains there, and I interpret this as a good indication that my touch is welcome. I feel self-conscious because this is the closest I've ever sat to Dorothy, and also the first time I have held Dorothy's hand for an extended period. I think that if we'd had more physical contact in the course of our relationship, this would be easier for me, now. At the same time, it was always obvious to me that being physically affectionate was not part of Dorothy's persona. The hugs that we did share later in our relationship were all the more precious to me because it took a long time for us to reach that level of comfort with each other.

I sit on the bed with Dorothy for almost an hour. Most of the time, I watch her face or our hands resting together on the bed. I listen to every breath that enters and leaves her body. I can hear when her breath deepens and I interpret this as Dorothy's body shifting into deeper states of sleep. I think about the description of the "death rattle" that was given at the hospice training, and I decide that it does not match the gentle snoring sound I sometimes hear. I hate the term! I still think there must be a better term for that phenomenon. It makes me think of cracking bones and snakes and the ancient, hooded image of the Grim Reaper. I think the term *death rattle* does nothing to demystify or alleviate my fear of death.

I bring my attention back to Dorothy's face and I wonder if she is conscious of my presence at all. I think about the many touching stories I've heard and scenes I've watched in films where people talk to their loved ones who are dying. I consider talking to her, but I realize that I always spent more time listening to Dorothy rather than talking, so it feels unnatural to just talk to her. Besides, I don't want to risk waking her if she is, indeed, asleep. I also have nothing I need to tell Dorothy, nor do I know what—if anything—she might need me to say to her. She may feel scared about dying, but even if she is scared, I know that's not the sort of thing that she would ever admit to me.

So, I continue to sit on the edge of the bed, watching Dorothy's face and our hands resting together, until it feels right to leave her room.

I stand, lean toward her a little, and then say, "Dorothy, I'm just going to out to talk to Terry and Len for a little while. I'll come back to say goodbye before I leave."

No response.

I walk out to the living room where Terry and Len are half-watching a talk show on television. Len is drinking a beer and smoking a cigarette. Terry must have lost her battle to keep him outside when he smokes. I try not to dwell on the fact that Len continues to smoke despite the fact that his mother-in-law is dying of COPD. I remember Emilia's little mantra, "Don't judge. Don't judge."

"So, how was your visit?" Terry asks.

"Well, I just sat and held her hand," I reply. "She's sleeping, I think."

Terry nods, curtly, and turns her attention to the television for a moment, her hand raised to her mouth in a nervous gesture—almost biting her nails, but not quite. I wonder where her thoughts have gone—to Dorothy, to what's ahead, to letting go?

"Did you tell her about the medicine?" Len asks.

Len's question wrenches Terry back to the present. She turns to me and says, "You know, we've been waiting for her medicine to come for 4 days."

I'm alarmed. "Which medicine?" I ask.

"Her morphine," Terry replies. "Although, we didn't tell her that's what it is. She's been having these bad pains in her legs, but I don't have anything to give her because we ran out this morning."

"So, what's the hold-up?" I ask. "Is there anything I can do?"

"I don't know what you can do that we haven't already tried," Terry replies. "You know, hospice has been a great service all along, particularly when we didn't need as much help. But I just don't understand why everything has to be so complicated now that we really need them."

I ask Terry to explain what happened. She says that Dorothy's doctor was supposed to write and fax a prescription to the hospice pharmacy, then they would deliver the morphine to Dorothy. The first prescription never came through the fax machine, and it has now taken several days to get another prescription written. The hospice pharmacy is now waiting for the doctor's office to fax the prescription so they can send the medicine. Meanwhile, Dorothy has run out of her previous order, and Terry is getting more frustrated by the hour.

As Terry finishes her story, the telephone rings. It's one of Dorothy's nurses, and I hear Terry say, "Okay, we'll call them again if you think it will do any good."

She hands the phone over to Len. "That was Marilyn. Could you call Dr. Smyth's office again? I can't deal with them any more."

Len crushes out his cigarette and leans forward in his chair with a look of determination on his face. The conversation begins civilly, but quickly degenerates. It's obvious to me that Len is being stone-walled by the receptionist; she is never going to let him speak to the doctor or to the medical assistant who is responsible for faxing the prescription.

Len's cheeks have started to turn red and his voice becomes strained. "Let me tell you something, I have no problem taking my mother-in-law out of your care and checking her into the hospital, today! You are, without a doubt, the worst, most uncaring, sons-of-bitches I've ever had to deal with! I don't know how you sleep at night ...."

Len has always appeared to me to be a shy and gentle soul. I find it touching that his concern for Dorothy has aroused him to this state of anger.

Len hangs up the phone and pushes himself roughly back into his chair, almost as if he is burrowing into a cave. He says, gruffly, "Now the medical assistant has gone out to lunch for the next hour. How long could it possibly take to put a prescription through a fax machine?"

My mind has started reacting to Len's announcement that they will put Dorothy in the hospital if they can't get any help. After all these months of taking care of Dorothy at home, I hate the thought that she could end up in the hospital. I wonder if Len and Terry even know what they will have to deal with if that happens.

I ask them, "Would you mind if I try calling hospice? I don't think you should have to deal with that doctor's office any more. Perhaps there's some other way they can get that prescription written?"

Terry sounds weary, "If you think it will do any good, go ahead."

I know that Dorothy's hospice team is in a meeting, so I tell the receptionist that it's an emergency and I need to speak with Dorothy's primary nurse. When Jackie answers the phone, I tell her that Len and Terry are still waiting for Dorothy's medicine.

"I've already talked with Terry this morning and told her I would handle it!" Jackie sounds exasperated.

"Well," I explain, "the other hospice nurse, I think her name is Marilyn, just called a few minutes ago and suggested that they call the doctor's office again."

Jackie sighs. "It sounds like a case of too many cooks in the kitchen," she says.

I agree. I didn't even know that another nurse was involved in Dorothy's case.

I continue, "Len called the doctor's office right away and they were very rude to him. I don't blame them for not wanting to deal with that office any more. Isn't there some other doctor they can access, through hospice?"

"But Dr. Smyth would have to sign off on any change of primary care physician, anyway," Jackie says. "I don't think it would be any easier getting him to do that than it has been to get the prescription."

I'm feeling more and more frustrated myself. I have to make her understand. I tell Jackie, "Len and Terry are ready to take Dorothy out of her doctor's care and admit her to the hospital so she can get her medicine."

"No!" Jackie exclaims. "That's a bad idea. Dorothy would have to be transported and admitted through the ER and then she might not even get the care she needs if they do that!"

"I understand what you're saying," I respond, glad that I seem to have her attention, "but Dorothy needs her medicine and I don't think Terry and Len need to be dealing with Dr. Smyth's office any more. It's not fair to them."

"You're right," Jackie agrees. "I'll call Marilyn and tell her we're going to handle it, then I'll call the doctor's office again. Could you let Terry know that I'm on the case and they won't have to deal with Dr. Smyth's office? I'll drive the medicine over to them myself as soon as the prescription comes through."

"Yes, of course," I say. "Thank you, Jackie. I'll tell them."

I feel bad for calling Jackie out of the meeting, but the thought of Dorothy ending up in the hospital makes me very anxious. Besides, I tell myself that I have never made a fuss about anything the whole time I've been visiting Dorothy. I figure I'm entitled to one little freak out, particularly when the change in her condition is so dramatic.

I turn to Terry and say, "Well, I suppose you heard most of that?"

"Yeah," Terry says, her mouth tense.

"I'm afraid I didn't accomplish very much," I apologize. "But Jackie says you don't have to call the doctor's office again, and she'll bring the medicine herself. I really think she'll be able to handle it and Dorothy will have her medicine soon."

Almost as if she has read my mind, Terry explains "Well, it's not like she needs it right this second, but I'm afraid that she'll come 'round this afternoon and she'll be in pain again and I won't have anything to give her." I see a flash of anxiety in her eyes and I realize that, for all her bravado, Terry is dealing with her own fears about Dorothy's death. I feel as though I want to give her a big hug and tell her everything will be all right, but I sense that would not be appropriate right now. Terry is just trying to do what she needs to do to get through each day and take care of her mother.

"I understand," I say. "I just want you to be able to concentrate on Dorothy and not have to be dealing with this kind of bureaucratic B.S."

"That's what it is," Len interjects. "It's just crazy that it has to be so complicated."

"You're right," I say. I consider leaving it at that, but I can't resist adding, "The snag in the system seems to be that hospice patients must have their own primary care physician, but those physicians do not work for hospice and are not paid by them. Where's their incentive for prompt service? That's why I was hoping that there might be some easy way for Jackie to change Dorothy to a hospice doctor, but she told me Dr. Smyth would still have to sign off."

"I know," Terry says. "Thank you for trying. I guess it's just been a long morning, and I always get upset when it seems like no one else cares about Mom."

I care about your Mom, I say silently.

I look at my watch. It's already well past the time I had planned to leave so I can make my next appointment. I walk back to Dorothy's room, take her hand in mine again and say, "Dorothy, it's Elissa. I have to go now, but I'll call again tomorrow. Goodbye." There is still no response from Dorothy.

As I walk to the door, Terry calls out, "I really appreciate all you've done."

I smile and say, "My pleasure."

Len walks me outside and says, "We did know about the doctor having to sign off. We were going to take Dorothy to the hospital and say that she wasn't in hospice and she didn't have a primary care physician so they would take her and give her the medicine. I don't take any bullshit from hospitals. I would have made them take care of Mom."

I smile and say, "Well, Len, I'm glad it's not going to come to that. I know that Dorothy would rather be here in her home. I'm sure Jackie will take care of it."

"Sure," Len replies.

As I drive away, my mind spins with disastrous fantasies of what would happen to Dorothy in the hospital. Of course, it could take hours for Dorothy to be evaluated by a physician and admitted. The physician probably wouldn't be trained in palliative or end-of-life care. The hospital would avoid giving her the morphine Len and Terry had wanted in the first place, because they'd be afraid to give Dorothy too much. And finally, Len and Terry did not want to tell them that Dorothy was a hospice patient, so the hospital would not know about Dorothy's DNR (Do Not Resuscitate) Order. I have visions of hospital staff shocking and intubating Dorothy's fragile body, then putting her on a respirator until someone (probably Terry) has to make the decision to take her off life support.

I shake my head in an unconscious effort to lose the images. That's *not* going to happen now. That's not going to happen.

"Thank you, God," I say to myself as I turn my mind back to my life outside Dorothy's place.

LETTING GO

The morning after my visit with Dorothy, I am only away from my apartment for a short time and I miss the call from my volunteer coordinator. A few weeks ago, a reorganization of LifePath meant that I was reassigned to a new coordinator, Roz, whom I met only once, briefly. It is a little before 10 a.m. when I pick up the phone and hear the dial tone that tells me I have a message. The electronic voice tells me that one new message was left at 8:41 a.m. Somehow, I already know what it will say.

"Elissa, it's Roz from hospice. Listen, dear, I'm sorry to leave this message on your voicemail, but I just got paged and I wanted you to know that Dorothy passed away. I'm going to be on the road now, but I'll be back in my office between noon and one, if you want to give me a call. I'm very, very sorry."

As I listen to the message. I feel as if something has wrapped itself around my body and I can't breathe properly. My throat constricts and I can hear my own pulse pounding in my ears. I pace across my tiny kitchen, taking two steps in one direction, then turning back the other way. I pick up the phone and put it down three times, before I finally burst into tears. I call my partner, Jay.

"I just got a voice mail message," I begin. "Dorothy died!" I cry.

"She did? Oh, Elissa! I'm so, so sorry," Jay says. "Do you want me to come over?"

"No, it's okay, really," I reply, surprised that I feel better already, just by hearing his voice. "I don't even know when she died or anything. I'm not even sure what I'm supposed to do."

"Are you going over there?" he asks.

"I guess so," I say, then my throat starts to constrict again. Tears fill my eyes as I say, "I'm really going to miss her, you know?"

"I know, baby, I know," he says. Jay really does know how I feel, and so I feel validated and comforted—exactly what I need right now. I'm so glad he is at home.

I promise to give him a call later, and decide to take a shower to calm myself down, but the falling water gives my body permission to open the floodgates and I cry in big, messy sobs until my eyes are burning. I get dressed and I try to pull myself together a bit, but when I look in the mirror, my eyes still look puffy and bloodshot.

Although I think I look terrible, I try calling Dorothy's place to see if I should come over. There is no answer, and I wonder if Dorothy could have died this morning, right before Roz called me. I know that Jackie would have gone to the apartment to pronounce Dorothy's death, but I don't know what would have happened after that or how long it might take. Basically, I don't know what's happening, and I don't know what I'm supposed to do. I need some guidance from hospice and I'm frustrated because Roz won't be available for another couple of hours. Besides, Roz only became my volunteer coordinator a few weeks ago, and she doesn't know about me and Dorothy. So, I call the one person who has always been there for me. I call Norma.

Norma's not immediately available, but I know she will return my call if I leave a message. I sit down at the computer as I await her call. Getting back to my writing, I feel as though I have flipped myself into another world. I'm calm, I don't feel like crying, and Dorothy's death could almost be the memory of a sad movie I watched last night, and not the real event that it is. I've settled right down by the time Norma calls me back.

"What's up, girl?" Norma says, her voice concerned.

My words spill over one another as I tell Norma about the phone message and my dilemma about what I'm supposed to do. I conclude by saying, "But I'm a lot calmer now than I was when I called you."

"Well, that's good," Norma replies. She tells me that it's appropriate for me to either call or just go over there. She says that there may be many things I can help with, and that I could offer to make phone calls or help with funeral arrangements, whatever they want. I feel as though I want permission to fall apart, but I also feel better, more in control, now that I have a role and a purpose. I thank Norma and head over to Dorothy's place.

When I pull up to Dorothy's apartment, Len is sitting outside with Sharon and two other people I don't recognize. The woman looks a lot like Dorothy, so I conclude this is her other daughter, Terry's sister, Connie. The man must be her husband, Chuck. From the collection of beer cans around their feet, Len and Chuck appear to have been drinking for some time. Len's heavy frame is slouching in the flimsy lawn chair, and he is looking at the ground. He seems lost, and I feel bad for him.

As I approach the group, Connie looks at me a little suspiciously, and I extend my hand immediately. "Hi, I'm Elissa, I'm Dorothy's hospice volunteer," I say.

Connie takes my hand nervously and blurts out, "She died."

"Yes, I know," I say, trying to reassure her. "That's why I'm here."

Len looks up. "I told them to call you," he says.

"Thank, you, Len," I reply. "I appreciate that. Roz, my volunteer coordinator, called and left a message this morning."

A second later, Terry appears in the doorway and says, concerned, "Did hospice call you?" She is holding a beer and quickly hands it to Chuck as she passes him on her way toward me.

"Yes, they did," I reply. "I'm so sorry, Terry." Tears begin to fill my eyes again.

Terry wraps her arms around me. It's amazing. We've never done more than shake hands, but it feels so right to hug her now, and I'm grateful for the contact.

"I know you are, honey," Terry says. She must sense the change in my breathing as my tears begin to fall, because she says over my shoulder. "Don't you get me crying now! Everything's fine."

I nod as she pulls away from me but keeps both hands on my shoulders as she looks at my face.

"You okay?" Terry asks. She opens another chair and places it next to her own. "Why don't you sit down?"

"Yes, thank you, Terry," I smile. "My volunteer coordinator left me a message this morning, but she didn't tell me what happened."

Terry and Len accept my implicit invitation to relay their story. Apparently Dorothy had continued to decline after I left yesterday, and Jackie, Dorothy's nurse, had visited briefly when she delivered Dorothy's medicine. Leslie and Sharon responded to Terry's suggestion that they come over in the afternoon. Connie and Chuck drove in from Miami and arrived in the early hours of the morning. Connie had woken Dorothy at around 6 a.m., and then at some time during the comings and goings in Dorothy's bedroom, Dorothy had simply stopped breathing. As I sit listening to the story, the various family members try to piece together the chronology, each one adding a detail or a correction to the facts. It occurs to me that I am witnessing the birth of a family story that will be repeated many times in the coming days and weeks.

A comfortable quietness settles on the group and my eyes wander to the trees that shade the breezeway where we sit. Dorothy loved sitting out here, and we'd spent countless hours sitting here together, watching the neighbors come and go, waiting for the mail truck to go by, talking about the weather or sitting in silence. I keep returning to the single thought, "She's gone. She's gone. She was here, and now she's gone."

My memories feel unreal. Now that Dorothy is dead, sitting here in the breezeway feels unreal. I feel like nothing is ever going to be as it was.

Terry reaches over and puts her hand on mine. "I want you to know that I appreciate everything you did for Mom." Connie looks over and smiles at me. "I know that Mom loved going out with you and I appreciate how much you cared about her."

"It was my pleasure," I say. "I looked forward to every visit, and I'm glad I was able to do something for her."

The family spontaneously shares some stories about Dorothy, and then begins to talk about funeral arrangements. Len says to me, "You'll come, won't you?"

"I would like to come," I respond. I feel very validated and supported, and yet I also know that I am not family.

After about an hour of quiet conversation, I sense it is time for me to leave. "I'm very sorry for your loss. Dorothy was a unique person; thank you for sharing her with me."

"Thank you, honey," Terry walks over and hugs me again. "Why don't you give us a call on Saturday morning? We'll know about the arrangements then."

"I will," I respond. "Take care," I say to the group as I turn to leave.

As it turns out, when I call on Saturday, I learn from Connie that Dorothy's funeral had been held the day before. Terry apologizes for not calling, and explains that there was some last minute confusion and changes to their plans. I tell her I understand. I know that I was not deliberately excluded, but I am very disappointed to have missed a chance to say goodbye to Dorothy. At the same time, the oversight drives home the fact that I am not, and never was, part of Dorothy's family. Perhaps this is part of what Norma meant when she reminded me to stay focused on my role as a volunteer.

Although I do visit Terry one more time at the apartment, that is the last time I see the family. Any grieving I have left to do, I realize, will have to be done in private.

ONE LAST TIME

A week after Dorothy's death, I decide to go down to the Crossroads Diner for lunch. It feels natural for me to go there after so many months of having lunch with Dorothy every week, and it also feels unnatural because I am going there without her for the first time. Perhaps I need my own ritual to say goodbye to Dorothy, but halfway down to the diner, I seriously consider turning back because I am having so much trouble choking back my tears. Every sign and storefront on the way to the diner reminds me of something that Dorothy used to say or do. It's hard for me to handle, but I feel compelled to go through with my plan.

I am glad that the diner is not crowded today. I quickly find a booth in the front and sit down.

Within a minute or two, Debbie walks up to the table with a glass of water and two menus.

"Are you waiting for Dorothy?" Debbie asks.

I've anticipated this moment, and I take a deep breath before saying, "You couldn't have known this, Debbie, but Dorothy actually died last week."

Debbie inhales sharply and her hand instinctively reaches for my shoulder, "Oh, no! I didn't know that. I'm so sorry."

"I know," I reply, "Thank you so much. I wanted you all to know because she loved coming down here so much."

"Well, you were a good friend to her," Debbie says. "I am so sorry. I'll let the other girls know."

"Thank you," I reply. I realize that these women, although they don't know my name, and are in every sense perfect strangers, they have also been the only witnesses to my ongoing relationship with Dorothy as we shared our weekly lunches. Most times we came here, it was just Dorothy and me, and these women saw us come here every week, so they know how much it hurts me to be sitting here alone.

"Can I get you anything, hon?" Debbie asks, gently.

"You know, I think I'll have the usual," I reply.

Debbie takes out her pad and pen, "Coffee, fish sandwich all the way, with a side order of fries. Coming right up," she says, and takes the menus away.

I remember how Dorothy used to get a kick out of the fact that the waitresses knew our orders, and would sometimes tease us about never trying anything new.

While I wait for my order to arrive, I look around the diner and think about Dorothy. At times, I have to distract myself and think about something else because I can feel myself start to cry, and I don't want to break down here in the restaurant. It is unusual and somewhat uncomfortable for me to eat alone in a restaurant. I feel even more uncomfortable to be sitting here without a book or a paper and pen to write with, unable to distract myself from experiencing my aloneness and my sorrow. I discipline myself to stay in the moment and appreciate the experience of being here, because I will not have another chance to do this. All of my emotions are a part of this experience, not just the happy ones, so I try to feel this as fully as I can.

I pay attention to the other customers in the diner. Although I don't recognize any faces, it's the usual crowd of clerks, trades people, and older folks from the neighborhood. I spot one older man who could easily be the reincarnation of Dorothy's "boyfriend," Don—a man in his 70s or 80s, quietly eating alone. I watch as the waitresses greet everyone with a smile, and address many of the customers by name. I consider the complaint I have often heard—that community no longer exists, and that nobody cares about anybody else. I realize that this diner was Dorothy's community. It didn't matter to her that the menu never changed, in fact, she liked it that way. What mattered to her, and what matters to me now, is that the women here knew her name, that this was a place where she could make memories, and that someone was always here to witness the quiet unfolding of her life.

This thought comforts me as I slowly eat my fish sandwich and fries. Every now and then, Debbie comes by and silently fills my coffee cup. It is the perfect combination of company and solitude. At one point, one of the other waitresses who often took care of us approaches my table.

"Debbie told me that Dorothy died," she says sympathetically.

"Yes," I reply, "It was last week. You know how she depended on her oxygen the last few times we came? Well, that was the beginning of a pretty rapid decline."

"I'm so sorry," she responds. "At least she didn't suffer for a long time," she says.

"You're right," I agree. "She was really only bedridden for a day, and then she passed away the next morning."

"Well, I just wanted to give you my condolences," the waitress says, briefly placing her hand on my shoulder.

"Thank you," I respond.

I finish my lunch and walk up to the counter to pay. Before I leave, I stand at the counter until Debbie can give me her attention.

I lean forward a little over the counter, and say, "Debbie, I just wanted you to know how much I appreciate ...." I start to lose my composure and my eyes fill with tears. The other waitress also turns to look at me, smiling her support. I take another breath and say, "Dorothy really loved coming here. Thank you for making this a special place for her."

"You're welcome, honey," Debbie says warmly. "I know you're going to miss her."

I nod, smile, and wave as I leave, unable to say any more.

As I start my car to drive home, a thought crosses my mind, and my tears begin to be punctuated with laughter.

I ask myself, what would Dorothy make of this scene? Of me sitting here blubbering in the car? She'd probably wonder what all the fuss was about. She would almost certainly question my decision to come here alone—very melodramatic! My heart still hurts, and I still feel very lost and strange now that she's gone, but I'm glad that thinking about Dorothy has made me take myself a little less seriously.

As I pull into Broad Street and head toward home, I think: "Well Dorothy, it turns out you were the teacher all along. Thank you."

10

Volunteers' Reflections on the First Year

The stories in this chapter are presented differently from the interviews presented in previous chapters because the form was generated from a series of group and individual interviews, rather than the single group interview that would have been ideal (see the Appendix for more details; see also Foster, 2005a). Because the stories in this third round of interviews speak to one another, and I trust that readers have a sense of the 6 volunteers and their stories up to this point, I have taken the responsibility of coordinating the voices here in a form that reflects the questions that I asked in the third round of interviews. This format is also intended to highlight some common themes among the responses, as well as the unique perspectives and relationships that emerged by the end of the year. Because my voice will dominate the final chapter of the book, it plays a less prominent role in the presentation of the following stories.

CATCHING UP

The first concern I had in the third round of interviews was to revisit the year and catch up on what had occurred in the 6 months since the second round of interviews. In the excerpts that follow, each of the volunteers I interviewed provides an overview of the year, and a description of their current relationships with their patients.

Tom shared the following summary. "I've been visiting in the nursing homes, and I've had two patients this year. Every time I went to see my first patient, she was worse. I'd go and she'd be curled up and she couldn't talk. The pain was so bad that I didn't feel like I did a whole lot. Then, I got my next patient, and he's also in a nursing home, but it's really old and there are a lot of homeless people there. When you pull up, the patients are out in the street, smoking in the parking lot. When you walk in, everybody's grabbing at you.

"I actually have Vicks in my car, and before I go in to visit my patient, I have to literally put it all over my nose. My patient's roommate has a colon problem—he goes to the bathroom outside of his body [he has a colostomy bag]. Sometimes I can't even go into the room. I've gone to visit a few times when my patient is sleeping, but there's no way I can stay, so I just leave and come back the next day. It's getting hot now so the Vicks is melting in my glove compartment. It's almost liquid, but I have to use it just to be able to stay in there.

"I worry that my patient will be taken off hospice, because there's absolutely nothing wrong with him that's terminal, except that he's a hundred years old. When she first told me about him, Patrice said she thinks his doctor or someone got him into hospice somehow, because he's all alone. He is really smart, really sharp. He remembers everything that ever happened to him. He'll remind me of things I told him 8 months ago that I don't even remember. He laughs and jokes. And he just turned a hundred about 2 months ago. He had a hundredth birthday party in the nursing home, and Patrice came with a bunch of hospice people. It was pretty cool.

"At the same time, he couldn't get any worse as far as his physical condition. He can't sit up; they have to crank the bed up so he can get up to the food tray. He can't get out of bed. They can't take him to the shower any more; they have to bathe him in the bed. He's in absolutely no pain, no medications, no diagnosis for being terminal. But I would think that if anybody fits the criteria for being in hospice, it would be him."

"So what do you think is in the future for you and your patient?" I asked.

"Even if they took him off hospice," Tom explained, "there's no way that I could stop seeing him. I'm the only person that goes to visit him, other than the social worker. When I leave, he's always asking, 'When will you be back?' and that sort of thing. Sometimes I get really busy at work, but I wouldn't tell him to hold off for a while. It just wouldn't happen. Now that I've heard that hospice reevaluates patients every 6 months, I'm getting worried."

Although Chris also volunteered in a state-run nursing home, Chris's experience of the year was somewhat different. He told me, "The place I'm visiting is really clean. It's a nursing home for individuals from very low economic backgrounds, but the people there cared a lot about them. It was amazing how clean it was, with none of the odor that is commonly detected in a lot of nursing homes. But it would be nice if people who reached that age could live like some of these other citizens I've seen, and be provided for in the way they *should* be treated.

"After the last time we spoke," Chris continued, "I had a few more visits with my first patient, and it pretty much went the usual way. I sat out on the patio with him, and we didn't really communicate. We made eye contact from time to time or smiled, but nothing spectacular happened. Then, Patrice informed me that he had gotten much worse, and I didn't get to see him any more. She said she would put me in touch with another patient. I wasn't given a choice at that point. I wasn't *attached* to my patient in any personal way. It didn't cause me, I guess you would say, *grief*, although I did feel sad for him. I didn't like that he had got worse, but then Patrice told me he was doing pretty bad all along. It seems like a lot of the patients don't appear to be doing quite as bad as they are. Now, with the second individual, the challenge is suggesting things that we could do together. I asked him, 'Would you like me to roll you out to the patio?' and he would not show any enthusiasm or even much interest in it. It was more like, 'If that's what you want to do, that's fine.' That didn't bother me, but it made me wonder whether this is something he really wants, or is he just saying this to please me. Even in good nursing homes, you have a lot of patients and few staff, so someone's needs will be neglected. Patients in that position have a tendency to not want to make any trouble."

Emilia has also been visiting patients in nursing homes. She explained, "My first patient was in her 90s. She had dementia but died of old age as far as I could see. She was sweet, but very demented. With my second patient, I showed up at the nursing home and she had been taken to the emergency room. She died and I never even got to meet her. My third patient, who is very sweet, has a heart problem, and I think she is also dying of old age, if she's really dying. I've been with her for about 4 months and she is in the same physical condition. Just about 2 weeks ago, I called Patrice to tell her that I'm getting married, and I'm buying a house, and I'm off to Brazil soon to visit my family, and I'm working in another town that's an hour away. So I said, 'I'm finding that I have to squeeze volunteering in, and that's not how I'd like to do it. I'd like to take some time off until July to get through this, and to be fair to my patient so that she gets someone, too.' I love my patient. When I leave, she tells me, 'I love you.' She's very with it. It's been great, but I'm no longer seeing her and she has another volunteer now."

When I asked how she felt about that, Emilia shared what had prompted her to take a break. She said, "I don't know what it is, but lately I've been feeling guilty and feeling pressured, and in part I know it's what's going on in my life. I have to stop and think that this is *volunteer* work. I came to hospice with the best of intentions, superexcited about getting a patient, with this fantasy of 'Oh, it's going to be so cool!' And now when the time comes to visit, what happened to that enthusiasm? It's a chore. It's in my to-do list. It sounds horrible, but I'm coming out of work and I'm thinking, 'Oh, I have to do hospice. Why did I volunteer? I don't even have time.' But this isn't hospice, this is my sweet patient that I'm talking about! This is playing in my head, and that's why I'm taking time off, obviously, but it's a major guilt trip.'"

Sarah described her year in the following statement: "I've been seeing the same patient since I started. She has congestive heart failure. Because of what I study, I've known ever since LifePath contacted me that she actually has around 7 years to live, which is average for someone whose heart is functioning at 50%. Her life is very full; she's not lonely. She gets calls from people every day; she has a *ton* of family! And that kind of makes me feel bad, because I feel I should be giving my time to someone who doesn't have all the people that she has. But then again, I get the impression that our conversations are very different from those she has with her family. Her daughter is great. They have a great relationship, but I never hear her talk to her Mom about her Mom. I almost feel like my purpose is to be the only person who listens to her.

"It is strange, though, to have a healthy, I mean, a *relatively* healthy, patient. Six months ago, hospice reduced her status, and she's up for evaluation again next week. I want to attend the team meeting and give them my view. They've spoken to her because they are 100% positive that she's going to be taken off the program. Outside of having congestive heart failure, she's really healthy. As long as she's in a wheelchair, she can do just about anything. She gets tired, but she's 79 years old, I think that's to be expected! Anyway, she has asked me directly, 'If they release me from hospice, are we still going to talk?' I said, 'Yes. I will continue to contact you. I'm not going to see you every 2 weeks, because I'm going to have another patient. But I will call and see how you're doing.'"

Shyanne also began visiting her patient in her home, then found she had to adapt to the changing circumstances and needs of her patient. She explained, "I was with my first patient for around 5 months until she passed away at the end of July. She had nobody, so even though she was taken off hospice while she was in rehab for a broken hip, I continued to visit her and I eventually became her health care surrogate. It was an extreme situation, but now that I look back, I did exactly what I felt I was called to do there. I maintained healthy boundaries. I know that when I went home after each visit, I detached from the situation immediately. I miss some of the conversations that we would have, but I truly don't miss *her*, because in terms of my life, she was always a hospice patient to me. It may sound cold and heartless, but she definitely is in her appropriate place in my heart and in my emotions. Although it was sad and it was difficult, I moved through her death pretty quickly."

Hannah was the last person I spoke to in the third round of interviews, and she revealed a dramatic change in her understanding and outlook in relation to her hospice volunteering. She told me. "My first patient died after only two visits, and I came to terms with that pretty well—but with my second patient, it was a whole different story. Miss Elliott, my second patient, passed at the beginning of January. After my second interview with you, Elissa, I experienced a change mentally and emotionally because of my own sickness and hospitalization at the end of the year. I was still as attached to her as I was before, but I had a different perspective on it. When I was in the hospital, I had all these people around me—my mother stayed with me—and yet I had this sense of loneliness. I'd wake up in the morning and be so grateful that somebody was there. I realized how crucial it was. I thought about all the patients, especially the nursing home patients who don't have someone there; it must be very scary.

"I didn't really understand Miss Elliott's death until I went through my illness in December. I realized that no matter how much I felt she had given me as a friend, what she received, however small it seemed, was much greater than I had ever imagined. I came to understand that everything was okay. I wasn't so scared any more, and it sort of made her death easier. The day that she passed, I wanted to see her, but I didn't. She actually passed during the time that I would normally go to visit. I think if I had been there, it would have been far more difficult. As it was, I know that there was nothing I could have done for her. She couldn't talk to me near the end, but I would talk to her. She stopped eating. She would drink a milkshake but that was about it. She lost a lot of weight. When she died, I didn't hurt as much as I thought I would. Once I knew that she was no longer suffering, it was more a feeling of happiness. I was also happy that I was able to provide that support for her."

These stories demonstrate the evolving experiences and shifts in attitude that accompanied the first year of volunteering. Although all of the volunteers except Sarah had experienced the death of a patient by the end of the year, and even Sarah was facing the imminent "loss" of her patient when she graduated, the meanings of those losses were different for each volunteer. Subsequent questions in the interview addressed specific insights associated with these experiences and also advice for other volunteers. Before sharing those responses, however, I present a unique experience that illustrates one of the roles that a hospice volunteer can perform in supporting a patient and family.

SHYANNE'S VIGIL

Although a number of us expressed interest in becoming what LifePath Hospice then called a "vigil volunteer"—subsequently called a 13th-hour volunteer—Shyanne was the only one in this cohort who had actually volunteered in this way. I asked her to share the story, and this is what she said:

"It was interesting seeing the goodbye process of the dad and the little girl," Shyanne began. "The patient was bed-bound, in a room at the hospital where she had worked for so long in the pediatric unit, and she'd actually been in a teaching position for many years. There was a steady stream of medical personnel coming in to say their goodbyes to her. Some of them were very tearful; some made jokes. There was no awkwardness, just sadness. They were losing their friend and their teacher. It didn't get emotional for me until the very end, because the little girl brought onion rings, which was her mother's favorite food. It was sad to see the child reaching out to her Mom with the onion rings. She was almost obsessive about it. She put them up on her mother's chest. By then, her mother was very close to death—you could see it, you could smell it, you could sense it—and she was just insisting on the onion rings, and she was mad that her mother wouldn't eat them. She didn't understand. When she had last seen her mother the night before, she was talking, and then 12 hours later, she went straight downhill. There were more drips and medications, there was more beeping, there were more people around the bed. So that was very tough watching the little girl, and knowing that her mother was dying.

"No one was saying those words to the little girl because they were afraid. Once those words come out, where do they go? How do you process them? And it was not my place. It was so hard. Part of me is saying, 'I'm trained to talk to these children. I know what to say.' But the parent in me said, 'Would you want a stranger talking to your child? Wouldn't you want to be the messenger?' My place was to be there for the patient. She had murmured a couple of times that she didn't want to be alone—'Don't leave me.' She didn't know who I was—if I was a volunteer, or a nurse, or her husband—she just held on very tightly to me. Then I left so that she could spend some time alone with her little girl and her husband, and she died within the hour."

"How long did you stay with her?" I asked.

"Hospice asked me to stay as long as I could," Shyanne responded, "and I was there for about half a day. It was all afternoon. I just felt that I didn't want to break the continuity. I remember that my stomach was growling at about 6 or 6:30. I remembered I hadn't eaten since breakfast, and thought that I'd better get home to my family. But my children were safe and cared for, and my only worry was that I hadn't eaten—big deal! I knew that I needed to be there and she would not let go of me because she didn't want to be alone. Her husband had stormed out in tears very early that morning because they told him that she was actively dying, and he left; he split," Shyanne gestures dramatically with her graceful hands. "He was gone for hours; they couldn't find him anywhere. It was late that afternoon or early evening before he came back.

"Initially, when he walked into the room, I was sitting there holding his wife's hand, and I had no uniform on, I wasn't in white, I wasn't a medical staff member. He looked at me; I put my badge on, stood up to introduce myself, and gave him my free hand. He couldn't really understand what I was doing there, and I just told him that hospice had called me, and it was part of my services to be with patients when the families couldn't.

"He said, 'Okay,' but he took a step back, and looked at his wife and his little girl with the onion rings saying, 'Mommy, Mommy, I've got your onion rings. You have to eat them; they're your favorite.' And he was just horrified—horrified at losing his wife. He looked like a deer caught in the headlights. He said, 'Are you coming back tomorrow?' And I said, 'If you need me, you can let hospice know, and they will contact me. You don't ever have to do this alone. That's why we're here.' So he sat down in the chair. He wouldn't even approach the bed.

"Her name was Nancy. And I think that Nancy had been in the position of taking care of him and their child for so many years, just the total nurse. He honestly didn't know how to handle seeing the tables turn and seeing Nancy be totally helpless, not being in the position of being in charge. He had to assume control, but he didn't even know how to control his own emotions, let alone the situation. And then the whole thought of raising a child alone, you could tell he was just ... overwhelmed. But so often, in a time of terrible grief like that, you're paralyzed. You almost need someone to hold your hand and say, 'This is what you need to do next.' But at that point, I just felt I needed to remove myself from the situation. I had done what I was asked to do for the patient, and she was not alone. I wish that I could have talked to the little girl, but that's her Dad's job."

I reminded Shyanne that she began volunteering for hospice to overcome a fear of death, and now she had not only witnessed the death of her first patient, Clarice, but she had also been present for this relatively young woman as she was dying. I wondered how this experience had affected her differently from Clarice's death.

Shyanne provided her typically thoughtful response. "The fact that Nancy and I were close in age made a huge impression on me. When I saw her little girl, I was thinking, 'Who would raise my children? They have their father but I'm their Mommy.' A few days later I was talking to my girlfriend about it and we chatted for about an hour, not about my patient, but as two mothers. Just talking about it really helped because we realized that, yes, it would be hard not having a mother, but our children would be fine. We were just thinking about that whole emotional, psychosocial, and emotional thing that children go through when they lose their Mommies, especially that little girl at age 11. She's just becoming a young woman herself, and you could tell she was close to her Mom. That was tough."

The story of Shyanne's vigil was important to include here because it provides an evocative account of an important role that volunteers can play in providing human contact and support, particularly when patients are referred to hospice in the last days or hours of their lives. This story is also important because it demonstrates that having a relationship history with the patient, while it is an ideal and can be significant to the work of the volunteer, it is not necessary to achieve the goal of making a connection and a difference in the life of the family and the patient. In the following section, I present responses to the question of what characterized the relationships between the volunteers I interviewed and their patients, particularly in relation to what they talked about, what they did together, and what this meant in terms of providing care at the end of life.

THE VOLUNTEER–PATIENT RELATIONSHIP

When I asked about the nature of communication in the relationship between volunteers and patients, Tom immediately addressed the issue of talking about death and dying. Reminding me of the time his patient mentioned he had been given the last rights, Tom relayed a similar incident that had occurred more recently. He told me, "My patient actually, right out of the blue, just looked at me one day, and asked me, 'Do you think there's really a heaven, or are people making it up to make them feel better?' The first thing I thought of was, okay, he's sick. He's letting me know that he thinks something is going to happen. I was trying to think back to the training, like, Was there a videotape on this?

"Anyway," Tom continued, "So I just said, 'Have you believed in heaven all your life?' He said, 'Yes.' And I said, 'Well, why would you stop now?' I just left it like that. It really threw me, because everything else we talk about is always football and politics, and all of a sudden, one of those questions that I was always worried about came right out of the blue. He didn't even work his way up to it!"

Sara described a very different response to similar moments with her patient. She explained, "One thing that I've never *ever* discussed with my patient is religion. She has absolutely no idea that I don't believe in God; she just thinks that I don't talk about it. She'll talk to me, but she's never asked me specifically what I feel. She'll tell me that she prays for me. Then there was this social event at her church for single people, and she tried to get me to go, but I said, 'I don't think that's such a good idea.' It's sort of interesting, because with anybody else in my life I would absolutely let them know my feelings. My family is very religious, and my

Mom jokes about the fact that somehow I can keep my opinions completely shut off with my patient, but with nobody else. And I'm like, 'Well, it's a completely different thing.' There's no reason for me to ever offend her that way."

When I asked if the relationships between volunteers and patients were like family or like friendships, Tom said, "My patient is a friend to me now. When the time comes, I'll probably be very hurt. I'm used to seeing him. It's like a part of my routine. I don't have to remember it; I just find myself driving over there."

Sarah's response echoed Tom's. "She told me recently, 'It's been good to spend time with you for a couple of hours, *as a friend*. I've gotten used to being able to talk to you, and share things with you.' It's nice for her to have someone to sit there and listen, about her husband, her kids, and her grandkids and great-grandkids. I recognize their pictures. I know who they are. I know her entire family structure—and she has a huge family. It's really interesting the way our relationship has changed over the year. For the longest time, we didn't touch each other much. But I've noticed more and more that she hugs me when I leave, and it doesn't at all bother me, but I'm not touchy by nature. It's funny that, without me really noticing, she just started doing it one day. It's something that she initiated and I don't pull back from. It's also a lot more personal than I thought it was going to be. She knows a lot more about me than I intended her to know, because she asks—and I never expected it to be that way."

Hannah also described being surprised by the friendship that emerged between herself and her patient, Miss Elliott. Hannah confessed, "I'd always thought of myself as a giving person, but I realized I was a lot more selfish than I thought because I was so worried about what the emotions were going to do to me. I realized that it's okay to feel that pain; I learned that from hospice, but I wouldn't have learned that if Miss Elliott hadn't come into my life. Even as I'm speaking to you now, I realize that it's had a huge effect on me. I know that the friendship my patient and I built meant more to her than I could feel at the time. I guess I learned that I have a lot more to learn! Miss Elliott would tell me sometimes that she thought the Lord wasn't taking her right away because He was saving her so we could meet and become friends through hospice. There were days when she was very tired, she was on oxygen, and when I got there, she would be asleep, but she would get upset if I didn't wake her."

I recalled that Tom went through the same experience with his patient.

Hannah continued, "Sometimes I would just go for a walk and come back in 15 or 20 minutes, but she didn't care, she would still get upset. That's when I first realized that it meant something to her. She would often tell me that she thought our purpose in our life was to help each other. I think she appreciated not only the companionship or the talks we had, but I think we had a *friendship*. It was as if I had known her for years, and I know that I was more than a volunteer for her. I think when you use the term *volunteer*, it seems so simple. But what we do in hospice, you can't possibly explain it just with the word *volunteers*."

Emilia responded quite differently to my question about relationships in hospice. It was clear from her decision to take a break from volunteering that she was in the process of revising her expectations. Emilia explained, "Maybe I was hoping to have a little bit *more* of a relationship with a person, but the setting just feels kind of cold. I'm not saying it was a waste, but I want more out of this, too. My patient now, we talk but she's never opened up. She never talks about her death or even about suffering. Maybe I just want to be touched. I hate to be selfish that way, but I feel very empty not having an identity. The nurses don't even know I'm from hospice; they just think I'm a granddaughter who shows up sometimes."

At this point in our discussion, Emilia became self-conscious of her negative tone.

"I'm so sorry I've been venting ..." Emilia said. "Actually, I'm glad you're doing this research, because I think I've finally realized what my problem was. I'm feeling detached. Lack of relationship with Patrice. Lack of relationship with my patient. It just felt weird because we all came in at the training and we did the little group photo and 'Here's your tee shirt!' and 'You guys are great!' But now, even Patrice doesn't really know who I am. It's like, I'm sending money, I'm donating time, but I'm not having any relationships. I think that my mother passed away and I wanted to see inside a person's head and be a part of that process. I don't feel like I'm a part of any process. One person was so old, she was demented, and she was ready to die. This one is also. And she calls me Linda! I'm not even me. So I think it's about detachment, and that might be interesting to look at somewhere in your research."

I am grateful that throughout the project, Emilia was willing to be honest about the challenges she faced in the activities of being a volunteer. Perhaps because most of us did encounter and enjoy relationships with the people we visited, it would be easy to overlook the ways in which a volunteer might come to feel disconnected and discouraged. Chris found similar challenges to those Emilia described because he also visited people in nursing homes who did not engage with him in conversation. Chris's response to his experience was different, however, and in the next section I share the advice he and the other volunteers suggested for people who may want to become volunteers.

ADVICE FOR VOLUNTEERS
AND HOSPICE-AS-ORGANIZATION

Chris responded slowly, in his soft, deep voice. "If someone can manage to visit a dying person at all, they need to concentrate on the importance of the human connection—concentrate on *being there*. The fact that someone is dying may be a source of extreme stress for the person who is visiting, and they may be trying to decide whether they even want to get involved. If they could see that being alone is worse than any feeling that they experience while visiting someone who is dying, then maybe they can muster the inner strength."

Chris elaborated on this idea. "I may not be able to remain totally unaffected by the fact that this person is dying, but it's not something that I can't do. It's not going to ruin me. So, even though we may not have any conclusive ideas on how to help, I think it's in the trying that it's really important. I think there's always a benefit in trying, even though you can't satisfy most problems. So, advice to the new volunteer would be to just understand why you're there. If you're really there to try to help, then don't let anything stop you from going in and helping. If you can't take it, then by all means get out. Hospice always makes a way for you to get out as easily as you got in—which is important."

Hannah's response echoed Chris's, and illustrated the change that had taken place between her second and third interviews. Hannah explained, "Before I got sick, I was focusing on what I would feel when Miss Elliott died, and afterward I was able to think, 'Well, she's here now, and I don't want her to be afraid, and if I can somehow alleviate that, then I will be okay with whatever happens.'"

Shyanne also reflected on the changes that had occurred in herself between the beginning of the year and the end. She told me, "If I were to look back to the beginning of the year, I think I would say to myself 'Just get out of your own way.' Spending too much time living up here in your head; and when you move down here into your heart, the gap between your heart and your head gets smaller as we get wiser, and softer, and gentler, with age and experience. You realize that when you get down to this place of thinking with your heart that your actions will all stem from love and wanting to do the right thing. When you move it up to your head—and you and Sarah as academics have to live up there a lot—it's a very safe place because you can make things make sense, but you can also scare yourself and talk yourself out of certain things. Maybe there are two pieces of advice I would give myself: Get out of your own way, and get out of your head."

Hannah expressed a similar idea. "Particularly if people are afraid of volunteering," she said, "I would say that any time you enter an emotional situation like that, how could you not feel fear? Especially with someone dying! At the training we were told, 'You are going to be given a patient who's going to die, and your job is to help with that process. You've had 16 hours of training now. You're ready! Go ahead. If you have any questions, just call me.' As a volunteer, you're in a position where there really are no guidelines. I think it's something that you have to go through the first time, then you realize that it's all in the time you spend, it's all in the relationship. Death and dying is a part of life. It's not like a separate mystical thing, and I don't think any amount of training can prepare you for that. Hospice does their best, but you still need that experience. It really is just someone coming into your life and you have to respond. So, I would tell people that whatever comfort you are able to give to patients, for whatever space of time, far outweighs any fears or worries that you may have."

Sarah summed up her experiences in the following way. "It's been an amazing experience for me. What's interesting is that my academic advisor tells everyone, 'I encouraged Sarah to volunteer for hospice so she could get some personal experience.' Then when I ask *him* about volunteering, he makes it sound like he doesn't have any time to do it. I work with all these professors who study the end of life, but don't come anywhere near people. And I've said to a lot of them, 'Why don't you do this?' And they say, 'I'm too busy. I have too much to do. I don't think I could handle that.' You spend your life researching people who are at the end of their life, but you won't take the next step to *be with* them? Really, all you're talking about can be as little as half an hour a week. If somebody is really, really sick, a half an hour is plenty of time, and it can make such a difference."

Shyanne also suggested: "The key to volunteering has to do with *being* in the moment, period: Being totally in the moment with your patient, and then leaving that moment, and being with your husband or your partner, being at home with your child, or telephoning a friend And totally allowing yourself to be with that person and to dance with that person emotionally, and *being there*, instead of future, past, maybe, ifs, what ifs, grocery lists, telephone calls, emails—letting all of that take a back seat to be in the moment with whoever you're with. I think it's a great philosophy for life, not only for your hospice patients."

During the interviews, I also invited the volunteers to offer advice for hospice as an organization.

Emilia offered the most feedback in terms of her relationship with the organization. She said, "I like Patrice very much, and at the training meeting, I was just enchanted, and thought, 'Wow. She's so great.' Then at the first support meeting, she said to me, 'Oh, Emilia, I know you're a vegetarian,' which I'm not. I understand that she's dealing with a thousand volunteers, but I remember having a conversation with her about my mother where she was so sympathetic. Then, she asks me the same questions over and over again, like, 'Your Mom passed away, right?' and that bugs me. Another time she compared me to another volunteer, and she said, 'Oh, Emilia, she reminds me so much of you. She's so young and shy.' Shy?! No, that's not me either! So, I started not liking support meetings, because for a minute there, I thought, 'It's so great to have a relationship with these people.' Now it's a turn-off. Patrice is great, but she doesn't remember a thing about me, so it all seems very superficial."

Tom also indicated that he felt some disconnection from hospice when he said, "There have been things that I was concerned about with my patient. I thought about writing questions about it on my patient notes, but I don't think hospice actually reads our progress notes. I'll write stuff on there, and nobody ever responds to it."

Sarah also said, "I send my notes in about certain things, but my coordinator will only call me once every 6 or 8 weeks or so, if she hasn't heard my voice. I don't know. It's like she calls just to check in on me, but I don't think she really cares. Like it's her job, but it's not something she really wants to do. My coordinator never knows anything about my patient, either, which bothers me. Every time, she asks me, 'What's your patient's diagnosis again?' And I'm like, 'No. She's *your* patient, actually.'"

I was reminded of my first interaction with Norma Sanchez, my volunteer coordinator, who told me that hospice is an organization like any other—it's not perfect. As one of the largest hospice organizations in the United States, with hundreds of volunteers, it is inevitable that even the small cohort of volunteers in this study would experience a variety of relationships with different members of the organization. Nevertheless, it is interesting to note the extent to which the volunteers (whether it was reasonable or not) expected a connection with the volunteer coordinators that echoed the connection the volunteers had with their patients. I counted myself fortunate to have worked for most of the year with Norma Sanchez as my coordinator, because she did give me the sense that she knew me, cared about me, and would be there whenever I needed her.

What is also remarkable in this advice to volunteers is that similar insights about the nature of hospice volunteering prevailed, and as evidenced by the comments in the section that follows, all the volunteers described having positive attitudes toward volunteering in the future.

LESSONS TO TAKE FORWARD

When I asked about whether she would go back after taking a break, Emilia explained, "I complain a lot, I know, but I still want to do this. I just think next time I'm going to try volunteering in the home because it's more like human contact, not that I don't have that with my patient, but—she called me Linda. I don't blame her, but she doesn't know my name. She hasn't got dementia, but she's definitely getting older and she'll say, 'Somebody came by today, from an organization called Hospital.' She doesn't even know. I know she needs me, she's so sweet and she needs the companionship, but I'm so busy and she doesn't even know my name."

Despite the challenges he found with the nursing home environment, Tom said, "I chose to volunteer in the nursing home because I was afraid of something happening to the patient when I was in their home alone. It seemed to me like almost everybody else in the training group had a medical background of some kind, and I have *zero*. So, I like knowing that all I have to do is yell out in the hall that something is wrong and somebody will come. I think I'll stick with the nursing home for that reason. At the same time, when I hear about other people's experiences, it seems it would be great to have a healthier type of patient, to be able to wheel somebody out to the street or to look at the trees or something."

Given the imminent graduation of her patient, I was interested to know what Sarah was going to do. "I'm going to continue seeing my patient as a friend," Sarah replied, "but not on the same weekly basis. I told my coordinator that I had no problem taking on another patient, but all along I've been seeing a very, very, healthy woman. That's why I never go to the support meetings that hospice offers. My patient is healthier than some members of my family! My coordinator said to me once, 'Well, maybe going to support would help you.' I said, 'Help me with what? My only issue with my patient is that she may not be my patient any more, and I'm not going to cry about that. I'm going to keep seeing her as a friend.'"

"I will continue to volunteer in the nursing homes," Chris told me, "because I feel like I've got something out of an experience if I go into the worst situations—and some of it is certainly despicable. It's very heart wrenching to see people in that position, but it helps me to feel. I'm not saying that everybody has to go to the worst nursing homes in order to feel that they're actually doing something. Everybody has needs regardless of their economic level. It's important to recognize when someone who's had it very good is not doing very well. I'm just saying that I'm one person who would rather spend my time trying to help the most needy."

Hannah spoke thoughtfully. "I came away from my experience with Miss Elliott feeling that, whatever I was doing, it was the right thing. Whatever comfort I was providing her, for whatever small duration, it was an important thing, much deeper than I had imagined. With my first patient, I wasn't sure I was really doing much. I picked up a new patient right away, but I never realized that I had made a difference. Now

that I realize that, I want to keep volunteering. I haven't taken on a patient since Miss Elliott died, but only because I'm still trying to recuper-
ate and I've been very busy at work, but I'm hoping to take on a patient
as soon as I can."

When I asked about lessons to take forward with us, Shyanne sighed
before saying, "Volunteering has been a really amazing experience
that's transcended anything I thought I would learn from it. The gift is
not the opportunity to volunteer, or not learning all these new things,
but it's truly the people, the patients. *They* are the gift, whether we see
them once or 10 times. It has also reaffirmed a lot of my faith in man-
kind. You can have dignity and have something to offer even when
you're dying and when you're older and when you're disease-ridden. It
really has blown whatever movie I had going on in my head as to what
death and dying looks like for me. It's like a director came in and just re-
did the movie, and that director just happens to be the hospice
experience."

"So what have I learned from hospice?" Hannah reflected. "I think
it's easier for me to provide comfort to other people who are going
through it. People feel that they can relate to you as a hospice volunteer
because you've been there, you see it. You may not be a family member
of a dying person, but you have been there."

Emilia took a different kind of lesson from her experiences in the
nursing homes. She spoke carefully and clearly, "Hospice is *wonderful*,
and I'm not quitting hospice by any means, but it's certainly been a reality check. For instance, there are things I didn't realize about nursing
homes. Every time I go, I get grossed out at the nursing home. I can't
help it. They don't take care of them! One time, there was puke on my
patient's pillow and nobody was cleaning it. That wears me out. I can't
wait to go home. I leave and I can breathe normal air, but I know I
shouldn't feel that way. This is a person. This could be me!

"I took my fiancé, Kevin," Emilia continued, "not so much to meet
my patient, but I wanted him to know. I said to him, 'We are never going
to do this to each other if we can help it. Period.' I don't see why it has to
be that way. I wish I had the opportunity to do more, physically, for
these people. It just disgusts me the way things are, but it's good to be
aware of what's out there. So, it's been a reality check. Every time I
leave, I'm more grateful for what I have; I'm more appreciative of what I
have. So maybe that's how hospice has helped me, so far."

Again, although Chris's experiences were similar to Emilia's, he
looked to the future with a different eye. He began with the observation,
"I used to hear people say that whatever doesn't kill you makes you
stronger. So, volunteering has sometimes put me in an awkward position, but I think that I may have learned how to work with people on an
even deeper level. As a funeral director, not only have I studied this, but

also just observation throughout my life—and this is no surprise to you, Elissa—death is a thing that we just *do not* deal with, or we deal with it improperly. We teach people systematically, especially young people, to be afraid of death. The Egyptians would be in as much contact with a family member during death as they would a newborn at birth. I think that would be something really great—to get people more aware of death and discussing death. I think that when you do, society will be a lot more compassionate. You'd have young folks growing up and wanting to preserve life, and not wanting to hurt people, because they would realize how precious life is."

With a similar attitude of hope, Shyanne looked back to the beginning of the year and then explained her new outlook on life and death. She affirmed, "I'm not saying that I relish the thought of dying, because I'm in love with being alive, but I'm also more at peace with the fact that with this life there will be an end. And when I think of my own death now, I don't get that choked feeling in my solar plexus. I still don't know how I will be when I am faced with it, but I know that when I think about it, I feel more peaceful and calm. I know that it's going to be out of my control, and there's a certain sense of safety in the act of surrendering that. I'm in a much more peaceful place, not only about death, but about life as well. And that's a wonderful thing for me."

I certainly feel that I have learned from all these volunteers and I cannot imagine having gone through my first year without the periodic sense making that occurred with the interviews. My heart echoed Shyanne's observation; I also felt a renewed faith in humanity that so many ordinary people, every day, are willing to do something that has turned out to be quite extraordinary.

Hospice and Communication at the End of Life

THREE ASPECTS OF THE VOLUNTEER'S JOURNEY: IDEALISM, CRITICISM, REALISM

Although this book is primarily dedicated to understanding the relationship between hospice volunteers and their patients, the three rounds of interviews I conducted over the course of a year allowed me to observe changes and developments in the volunteers themselves, specifically their attitudes toward hospice as an organization, and their understanding of their role in providing end-of-life care. For volunteers and prospective volunteers, and for those who work with them, the following observations are intended to provide a vocabulary for talking about the ways that volunteers' attitudes may shift over time. As in the reflections at the end of chapter 8, I return to the concept of dialectic tension to describe the dynamic relationship among hospice volunteers, the work that they perform, and the hospice organization.

Although the volunteers' experiences were highly diverse, I noticed striking similarities in the issues and questions we raised during the course of the first year. At various times, our perceptions shifted in relation to our roles, our relationships with patients, and our understanding of hospice as an organization. I refer to these perceptual shifts as *aspects* of the volunteering experience, to distinguish them from the linear concept of stages or phases. The word *aspect* has two related meanings, both of which are relevant to this discussion. The first connotes a dimension, side, or characteristic, and the other connotes an outlook or perspective. For the purposes of aesthetic balance and conceptual simplicity, I refer to these three aspects of the volunteer experience as *idealism, criticism,* and *realism.*

Although I describe the three different aspects as corresponding to the three rounds of interviews—directly after the training, 6 months later, and at the end of a year—I do not intend these to be strict categories that describe the volunteers' development at each of those stages. Rather, I present them as a description of the changes in attitude we generally experienced as we progressed on the journey, each in our own way and in our own time. Furthermore, within a volunteer's single telling of an experience, it is often possible to identify all three attitudes or aspects—idealism, criticism, and realism—as the volunteer's outlook or understanding changes through the telling of the story.

During the first interval of the research project, the volunteers' stories were marked by feelings of idealism as we entered hospice, became part of the hospice culture, and experienced our first visits with hospice patients. Even before I walked through the doors of LifePath Hospice on the first day of training, I was motivated to volunteer by events in my personal history and my desire to understand relationships at the end of life. The histories and motives of the other volunteers may have been different in their detail, yet we all came to hospice knowing that the basic activity of our volunteer work would be to visit with and offer support to people who were dying. Informally, Emilia, Tom, and Hannah told me they did not generally disclose to other people that they volunteer for hospice, partly because people tended to respond with the backhanded compliment, "Oh, hospice! I don't know how you can do that. It's so sad." Because death is stigmatized in our culture, most people would rather not think about dying at all, and so they did not know how to respond to news that someone was a hospice volunteer. In contrast, the volunteers were not "turned off" by the idea of visiting with people who were at the end of life, and those of us who were fearful—like Shyanne and I—recognized our fear as a state of mind or emotional reaction that we desired to challenge and overcome. Nevertheless, understanding and believing in the goals of hospice care are not sufficient motivation to actually sign up, complete the training, and stay for a year. Each volunteer was compelled to commit to hospice by something more personal, moral, or central to his or her identity.

One sentiment that was expressed on several occasions by the volunteers was the desire to "give something back" to society, as Emilia, Tom, Shyanne, and Hannah each phrased it. Chris and Sarah viewed volunteering as a response to a recognized social need related to aging. Without exception, we all saw volunteering as an ethical responsibility, and many of us had volunteered for other organizations. For me the idea of becoming a hospice volunteer contributed to my identity as a socially responsible and moral person. I propose that, particularly at this early stage of our volunteer work, idealism characterized our belief in hospice and our faith in our own ability to affect the lives of others positively by contributing our time, energy, and goodwill.

Idealism, in a different sense, was also evident in our unrealistic expectations and projections about what volunteering would be like. My idealism about hospice translated into a sense of heroism about my role as a volunteer, which was simultaneously undermined by the doubting voice that told me I would not be able to "do it." In his first interview, Tom revised his fantasy of talking with hospice patients about some of the books he had read about death and dying, because once he began visiting his patient he realized "that's the opposite of what I should be doing." Similarly, Emilia confessed to thinking that she might have a patient who was interested in hearing some of her stories, until she began visiting a patient with dementia who couldn't remember her name and often appeared to be in another world.

In addition to our personal ideals and projections, our training sessions also socialized us into the hospice version of our roles and goals. Our idealism about hospice was demonstrated—particularly in the first round of interviews—by our unconscious adoption of the hospice language, a sign that we had begun to internalize hospice values regarding death and dying. In addition to using the term *patient*, (a label that was never questioned by the volunteers or the hospice professionals) some of the phrases that turned up repeatedly in our conversations include: "it's not about you, it's about the patient"; "my patient took a turn for the worse"; and "making a difference." We also began to use terms such as *actively dying*, and we described monitoring our *boundaries*.

Despite being told by our trainers that there was "no right way" to be a volunteer, many of us left the training with a sense that there *was* such a thing as the "ideal" volunteer–patient relationship. We faced our first visits fearing that we did not know enough. As we entered the world of the volunteer–patient relationship, our idealism continued. I remember feeling a sense of nervous excitement when I first visited Dorothy, much like the feeling of a first date. I was hyper-conscious of every communicative choice I made, trying to do and say the right thing. I also sensed that because Dorothy and I didn't know much about each other, there was a possibility that we could have an ideal relationship—there was no painful history, no negative information, and every reason to feel optimistic. When the situation was less than ideal, as it was for Emilia, Chris, and Shyanne, they found ways to construct the volunteer–patient relationship as significant because of the kinds of challenges that it represented. Shyanne, a white South African, found meaning and opportunity in accepting her first patient, who was an African American woman living in the projects. Of his patient, Chris said optimistically, "Perhaps I will learn how to care for someone who doesn't talk to me."

Hannah said when she volunteered for a patient who reminded her of her fear of dying alone, "it was exactly what I needed."

The idealism of our initial days in hospice gave way to criticism, in the sense that we started to question some of the assumptions of hospice volunteering, particularly with regard to the volunteer–patient relationship. Six months into the first year, some volunteers showed signs of breaking away from conformity to hospice rules. We resisted the guidelines that we had been taught during our training. This resistance emerged particularly when hospice policies and procedures threatened our relationships with our patients. For example, when Tom suspected that his patient did not fit the category of an appropriate patient, he decided that he would continue seeing his patient after he was taken off the program. Although we were taught that volunteers are only supposed to visit patients as hospice volunteers, Tom quickly felt a commitment to his patient that precluded an end to their relationship on the sole basis of a hospice regulation. The important issue that Tom's struggle exposes—which I discussed at length at the end of chapter 6—is the distinction that hospice must make under Medicare between providing care for dying patients versus care at the end of life. As relatively free agents, the volunteers made choices about how to respond to the needs of their patients independent of hospice definitions and guidelines. Shyanne not only continued to see her patient during a period when she was not in the program, she also became her patient's health care surrogate. In this case, Shyanne's sense of personal responsibility and social justice overruled the prerogatives of hospice as an organization—though she clearly conformed to the philosophy of hospice care.

The criticism aspect of the volunteers' experience also reflects the problems we encountered with the canonical story of the volunteer–patient relationship, which we had absorbed during the training. Essentially, some of us began to sense that "my relationship with my patient doesn't fit"; "I'm getting too close" ; or "I'm not doing enough to help." In Hannah's relationship with her patient, Miss Elliott, feelings that she was "not doing enough" as a volunteer actually masked a deeper concern. As Hannah thought about helping Miss Elliott come to terms with death, she realized that she was having trouble accepting that her patient was going to die. As a normal consequence of bonding with a hospice patient, this conflict poses a serious dilemma. Because I had grown close to Dorothy, this question became significant for me too, and most of the second interview with Hannah was devoted to this topic. Of course, we did not "resolve" the dilemma because what we faced was the pull between our growing attachment and our fear of loss—a quintessential dialectic of the volunteer–patient relationship that I discussed at the end of chapter 8.

After we had lived through the experience of volunteering, the third round of interviews were marked by an attitude of realism about our role, our relationships with patients, and the strengths and limitations of hospice as an organization. None of us felt particularly heroic. We also recognized the truth of what Norma had told me months before the project began: "Hospice isn't perfect." We had learned to live within the duality of enjoying our patients in their life and accepting their deaths. We had learned to accept the duality of hospice as an organization that transcends many problems of modern dying, while it remains a bureaucracy with flaws like any other. We had also learned to accept our own limitations regarding what we could do to make a difference in our patients' lives. Perhaps most importantly, we had experienced what it meant to develop a relationship with someone at the end of life, and through facing the illness and deaths of our patients, we shed many of the stereotypes and assumptions that we had started with.

As Hannah described it, her own illness and hospitalization constituted an epiphany in her understanding of her role. Several months before her patient's death, she had been afraid that she was not doing enough, that she was becoming "too attached," and that she did not want to experience the pain of her patient's death. After her own hospitalization, Hannah realized the value of what she had provided by being with her patient, which in turn comforted her when her patient died. Hannah experienced the pain of loss, but it was "not what she thought it would be." Emilia's change in perception had more to do with the organization and the nursing home environment than her interactions with patients. By the end of the year, Emilia described how she lost her illusions that hospice would provide personal connection and a kind of family for her. She also learned that the nursing home environment presented a substantial obstacle to her ability to connect with patients. Emilia realized that to continue as a hospice volunteer, she would need to rely on her own desire and exercise her own agency to choose the environment in which she could feel comfortable enough to enjoy being with her patients.

I reiterate that the concepts of idealism, criticism, and realism describe general shifts in the volunteers' perspectives over time rather than strict developmental stages; however, I deliberately presented these three aspects of the volunteers' stories in terms of how they corresponded to the three intervals of the research project. The impact of time is an important factor in relationship research, particularly for those who adopt a relational perspective that emphasizes development, process, and change (Duck, 1990), as I do. This approach also appealed to me because it retained the sense of plotline that is a crucial aspect of narrative and storytelling. The naturalistic drama of the *well-made play* is presented in three acts, and the traditional Western narrative has at its core an inciting incident, which rises to a climax, followed by a denoue-ment (Esslin, 1987). Kerby (1991), a narrative theorist, suggested that human experience is similarly organized in terms of time. He observed, "experiences come to one not in discreet instances, but as part of an on-going life, my life" (Kerby, 1991, p. 16). What this means for volunteers in this study is that we made sense of our experiences not as isolated in-cidents, but based on what had happened to us before, both with our patients and in our lives outside hospice.

As I described in chapter 8, dialectical approaches to understanding relationships (Baxter & Montgomery, 1996; Montgomery & Baxter, 1998; Rawlins, 1992) also constitute a time-conscious approach to the study of relationships. In particular, Conville (1998) proposes a helical model of relationship changes that combines both a dialectical and a de-velopmental perspective. Conville's approach is also grounded in a nar-rative approach to relationships; he suggests that stories reveal phases of security, disintegration, alienation, and resynthesis as relationships transition from one developmental stage to another. In essence, Conville's model depicts movement between an acceptance of the rela-tionship as it exists, through a period of questioning and rejection, and a return to acceptance, albeit of a revised relational form or of a new un-derstanding of the relationship. Similar developmental phases have been found in the communication of small groups as they move from a phase of group formation, through conflict, to the emergence of group norms (Brilhart & Galanes, 1995; Rothwell, 2001). Also at the level of in-stitutions such as hospice, social theorist Archer (1995) describes three parallel phases within structural elaboration, as social institutions move from stability through instability, and back again to stability, once a new structure has emerged. Relating these theoretical perspectives back to the volunteers, I perceive our development as similarly cycling through attitudes of acceptance (idealism), questioning or rejection (criticism), and returning to acceptance, with a revised understanding of ourselves in relation to our volunteer roles (realism).

In proposing these terms to describe the volunteer's journey, I em-phasize that the attitudes and relationships of the volunteers to hospice are subject to the same kinds of fluctuations and dynamic interplay as other kinds of relationships. Part of the idealism that characterized our early days included the notion that we should strive for the right atti-tude or approach to the hospice work. Although most of us achieved a level of comfort and stability (or realism) by the end of the year, it is im-portant to recognize that part of the volunteer's work depends on pas-sages of idealism when we become reinspired by the hospice vision, and also times where we express criticism of practices or interactions that do not match this vision. Being able to put language to these shifts in atti-tude may help volunteers and those who work with them to notice when they are occurring, and to accept all three as important to the experience of volunteer work in hospice.

HOSPICE VOLUNTEERS AS ANTIDOTE
TO THE PAIN OF SOCIAL DYING

In this section, I return to the questions that prompted my study in the first place; namely, how we can best communicate with people who are dying, and what is the unique contribution that volunteers make to the holistic care that hospice provides. I will begin by addressing the second question, because its answer frames and supports my conclusions about communication at the end of life.

The hospice patient exists in what anthropologist Turner (1995) calls a liminal space (literally, a threshold) between the point at which their terminal status is decided and the moment they die. Seale (1998) describes this time as a crisis because it creates feelings of individuation and that one is "falling out of culture" (p. 25). Seale's (1998) phrase refers to the experience of losing social contacts—a shifting consciousness of time, personal stigmatization, and an estrangement of the body created by physical pain and other symptoms, all of which create disconnection, disharmony, and disintegration (Carr, 1995). The sum of these experiences is encapsulated in the idea that there can be a social death (Lawton, 2000; Seale, 1998) that precedes physical death. In chapter 6, I indicated that dying could be framed as a social as well as a physical process, and the concept of social death refines this idea by focusing specifically on the "loss of self which stem[s] from a loss of relationships" (Lawton, 2000, p. 148). Although the term *social death* was not used during the hospice training to define our role or describe our contribution to the care of the patient and family, it helps to explain why the volunteer–patient relationship plays an important role in end-of-life care.

Lawton's (2000) analysis of social death was grounded in an ethnographic study of a nursing home, and focuses on extreme cases of isolation in which one could say that the patient had, in a sense, already died because they had outlived or exhausted all social contacts, or no longer influenced the lives of people they cared about. This was the case with only a few of our patients, most notably Chris's patients and Tom's first patient. Although this kind of isolation was rare among the small number of volunteers involved in my study, debilitation associated with a prolonged illness, the isolation resulting from placement in a nursing home, and the stigma of approaching death can all contribute to shrinking a hospice patient's world. Such shrinking may not constitute a complete social death, but it can be understood as perpetuating the process of social dying, which has its own associated pain. If the volunteers' primary goal is to engage in an interpersonal relationship with a patient, I propose that the volunteer role is designed to address and alleviate the pain associated with social dying.

As my conversations with Chris suggested, the need to address a patient's social death almost certainly derives from our horror at the thought that anyone would die alone. Beautifully illustrating this idea, actor Steve Martin (2002) described his responses to his father's death in an essay published in *The New Yorker*. Here is part of the final paragraph:

> My father's death has a thousand endings. I continue to absorb its messages and meanings. He stripped death of its spooky morbidity and made it tangible and passionate. He prepared me in some way for my own death. He showed me the responsibility of the living to the dying. But the most enduring thought was expressed by my sister. Afterward, she told me she had learned something from all this. I asked her what it was. She said, "Nobody should have to die alone." (p. 87)

The idea that it is terrible to die alone has a taken-for-granted quality; thus, I explore briefly how this idea affects the construction of the volunteer–patient relationship. Two ideas in Martin's concluding passage relate to social death and the role of hospice volunteers. The first idea is suggested by the expression "nobody should have to die alone," and the second idea is that we all have a responsibility to support those who are dying. Rather than saying, "nobody *should* die alone," Martin's phrase incorporates the idea of a person's choice or preference. As I attended hospice support meetings during the course of this project, I occasionally heard stories about individuals who repeatedly refused volunteer visits and also made it difficult for hospice personnel to enter their homes to provide care. In these cases, hospice would provide what services they could while respecting the wishes of the patient. One could surmise that for these patients either a social death had already occurred, or they simply preferred to live and die alone. During the course of my volunteer work, I delivered groceries to a woman who was dying of cancer, alone and in an almost bare apartment. When I commented on her need for a volunteer, Norma told me, "She's determined to do this on her own." Interestingly, these cases do not provoke the same feelings of horror or pity as situations where a person is dying alone, yet *desires* social connection, support, and validation. When the volunteers assessed the value of their work, it was the second type of patient, the one who desired social contact, whom they regarded as the most ideal partner for a volunteer–patient relationship, and the one who would benefit most from hospice.

This brings me to the second idea—that we have a responsibility to those who are dying. As I suggested earlier, the volunteers come to hospice with a sense of social responsibility and are motivated to devote their time and energy to a worthwhile social goal. That they choose to volunteer for hospice also means that they believe in the importance of supporting someone who is dying, partly for the sake of the individual patient, but also because of a more generalized belief in the value of a human life. When I talked with the volunteers about how sad or how terrible it was to think of someone dying alone, the particular characteristics of the individual mattered less than the fact that a human life was ending without anyone there to witness and care. For example, in my first conversation with Norma, I felt a deep sorrow when she told me about the only patient for whom she had been unable to find a volunteer—a man who had been convicted of child sexual abuse. Despite the offensive nature of his crime, I found it hard to accept that no one would volunteer to visit him. I disliked the idea of anyone dying alone, and I did not like the implication that I was a member of a society that would abandon someone when they needed connection and support. Also embedded within my emotional response is the belief that human life is more precious when someone has little time left to live.

As demonstrated by many of the stories in this study, the volunteer–patient relationship can be an affirming response to social dying. This may be the fundamental finding of my study, and a substantial feature of hospice as a humane alternative to dying in a hospital. Even in situations where our patients had family or friends involved in their lives, the physical aspects of deteriorating health and the burdens of caregiving could become obstacles to social relationships, particularly of the kind that validate dimensions of patients' lives outside their illness and process of dying. Sarah's patient was embedded in a network of strong family relationships and friendships. Sarah understood her contribution to her patient as someone who "doesn't talk constantly about what [my patient] is feeling or what she's doing, and doesn't harp on her about what she ate the night before and did she cook or not." In Dorothy's case, she lost her husband, then the companion she met at the diner, and she lost her autonomy when she could no longer drive—all these losses contributed to shrinking her social world. Although at first I resisted the idea of driving a hospice patient anywhere, my outings with Dorothy became a precious experience for me, because they allowed her to be herself and reconnect with the world in a way that she couldn't at home.

The concept of alleviating the pain of social death resonates with a body of research related to *social support*, which has been studied from sociological, psychological and communicative perspectives (Burleson, Albrecht, & Sarason, 1994). Social support can be defined in a variety of ways; however, a communicative perspective suggests that supportive messages, exchanged within specific relational contexts, can contribute to, and in some ways are essential to, emotional and physical well-being. Although many studies of social support examine the presence or absence of explicitly supportive messages, or types of supportive messages in various contexts, Barnes and Duck (1994) argue that everyday exchanges within relationships implicitly constitute support. Rather than focusing research attention on those messages that are intentionally and obviously "comforting," or "helping," Barnes and Duck (1994) suggest a broader scope for analysis that includes any symbolic activity that "communicates implicitly the value of each person to the other" (p. 178). It is this broader conception that most reflects the function and characteristics of the volunteers' communication with hospice patients.

In earlier chapters, I reflected upon different manifestations of dying as they function in the context of volunteer–patient relationships in hospice. In chapter 5, I discussed the impact of physical processes of dying and in chapter 6 I examined the construction of dying as a category that is used to manage enrollment and graduation from hospice. Social death is a third manifestation of dying that can help to explain the function of volunteer–patient relationships in hospice care. Hospice volunteers negotiate their patient's physical dying so they can respond affirmatively to the pain of their social death, and establish a relationship that often transcends the definition of dying to which hospice is expected to adhere. Communication is central to the relationship between hospice volunteers and patients. Specifically, if the concept of social death helps to explain *why* the volunteers entered and maintained these relationships, as well as *what* we believed we were achieving through them, then communication is *how* we constructed the relationships, through the tangible, everyday activities that we shared with our patients.

Research has shown that "final conversations" perform important relational functions between caregivers and people who are dying by generating meaning and providing a sense of closure (Keeley & Koenig Kellas, 2005). There were very few examples of such final conversations or direct communication about dying in the volunteers' accounts, which perhaps illustrates an important distinction between caregivers and volunteers. For example, during her second interview, Hannah became concerned because her patient did not talk about concerns related to dying. As Hannah put it, "I don't see any of the issues [about dying] we discussed in hospice training. Instead, we talk about whatever she wants to, which sometimes is nothing." Because our relationships began when (and because) the patients were given a terminal prognosis, we did not have the same need to discuss dying or to achieve closure on our relationships with our patients. Nevertheless, there were many examples of statements from the patients that helped to define and give meaning to the volunteers' relationships. In her third interview, Hannah described how her patient "would often tell me that she thought our purpose in our life was to help each other," and Sarah's patient told her, "It's been good to spend time with you for a couple of hours as a friend." These statements suggest that one of the functions of final conversations, "(re)constructing relational identity" (Keely & Koenig Kellas, 2005, p. 377), does occur within these relationships when patients explicitly express what the volunteers' companionship has meant to them. I know that I felt appreciated each time Dorothy ended our visits by saying, "I enjoyed it, honey. I always do, you know."

As I described at the end of chapter 7, the few examples where direct communication about death did occur tended to be framed in a way that minimized the centrality of dying to the volunteer–patient relationship. For example, Dorothy shared her philosophy about dying on two occasions when she told me, "When The Man Upstairs calls your number, there's nothing you can do about it," but it was never a central feature of our conversations. Tom's patient told him one day that the priest had been by to visit, then commented, "He gave me my last rites. Do you think they're trying to tell me something?" These examples stand in contrast to the kinds of philosophical or spiritual discussions about dying that were the substance of my media-influenced fantasies during the training.

Before concluding this discussion about the absence of conversation about death and dying, I should briefly return to one story in which such conversations took place between Shyanne and her patient Clarice. After Clarice had been admitted to an ALF for rehabilitation, she was taken out of hospice for a period of time during which Shyanne continued to see her and accepted the role of Clarice's health care surrogate. Shyanne brought with her the well-developed relational skills and perspectives of a counselor, which may be why she had the confidence to enact her relationship with Clarice in ways that did not always fit the hospice story we had been socialized into through our training. At first, Clarice would not talk about death, but when Clarice's cancer advanced to a point where she started to deteriorate rapidly, Shyanne actively pursued lines of questioning that would help her to understand Clarice's needs and wishes. As Shyanne said, "I *needed* to talk about it." Because of the role that Shyanne accepted in Clarice's life as her health care surrogate, Shyanne became more like a family member to Clarice, which appears to have given her the freedom to initiate conversations about death and dying that the other volunteers couldn't or didn't.

Extending the discussion from chapter 7, in response to Seale's (1998) contention that hospice relies on conversation as central to "the good death," I have shown that this did not appear to be true in practice—certainly not for the volunteers. A related element of Seale's (1998) critique of hospice is that the concept of growth at the end of life (Byock, 1997; Kübler-Ross, 1986) inherently privileges a psychological view of the self (Lawton, 2000; Walter 1994). This criticism posits that an inherently Western (Lawton, 2000) and individualistic view denies the body as a "key player" in end-of-life relationships, and fails to recognize the ways in which the self is relationally and intersubjectively constructed. Morris (1998) offers a qualitatively different interpretation of hospice. He suggests that in hospice "the dying patient is the focus, of course, but the patient and family *together* (including extended and non-traditional families) constitute the basic unit of care; personhood extends beyond the skin" (Morris, 1998, p. 239). Morris's observation reflects the importance of supporting the relationships of the person who is dying, which corresponds to the idea that hospice care addresses the social dying of the patient in addition to bodily and psychological deterioration. Within the hospice team, the purpose of the volunteer's work is to engage in a personal relationship with their patient, to get to know them through regular and ongoing interaction.

Although Western individualism and psychology may undergird hospice-as-philosophy, my observations suggest that hospice-as-experienced is fundamentally *relational* and not individualistic. Furthermore, the act of *being with* a patient acknowledges the importance of *bodily presence* over psychological understanding. As I will describe in the remainder of this chapter, the very nature of the relationships in my study relied on intersubjectivity (Bruner, 1986)—which can be simply understood as the implicit and intuitive dimension of communication, as well as a meaningful degree of blending between self and other (Laing, 1990). This blending was not a matter of interpersonal boundary transgressions (a psychological construct), but rather an extension of the relational context in which communication at the end of life occurs.

My work with hospice was motivated originally by my desire for personal growth, but after the volunteer training I understood that my role needed to be primarily responsive to the patient's and family's needs, not my own. My earlier analysis of the interaction between volunteers and patients suggests that *what* is talked about is relatively insignificant in terms of establishing the meaning of the hospice experience. Far more crucial is the role of intersubjectivity, through which volunteers and patients make sense of their relationship and the connection they have with one another. If one accepts, as I do, that human beings do not operate from a basis of objective cognition, but rather through a process of subjective interpretation (Varela, Thompson, & Rosch, 1991), then it is what we feel emotionally and interpret intuitively that tells us how to proceed in the volunteer–patient relationship. In each of the stories presented in this study, common sense, or *embodied cognition* (Varela, Thompson, & Rosch, 1991), played an implicit and central role in the ways the volunteers communicated with patients.

The contemporary discipline of interpersonal communication is grounded in the work of theorists such as Bateson (1951) and Laing (1990), who highlight the function of intersubjectivity in establishing and maintaining patterns of relationships. Bateson proposed that messages operate on two distinct levels, the report and the command, which Watzlawick, Beavin, and Jackson (1967) later termed the *content* and *relational* levels of messages. According to this distinction, in addition to the basic information conveyed by its manifest symbolic content (language and ideas), a message also conveys tacit information about the relationship between or among the communicators. Laing (1990) refers to this as the *implicit* level of communication, at which the meaning of a message is interpreted according to inferences about what was *intended* by the speaker. The activities that the volunteers performed, the topics we discussed, the fact that we were not paid, even the most basic act of visiting our patients regularly, all conveyed implicit messages about our commitment to our patients and their value to us.

Particularly during the early stages of our relationships, the hospice volunteers paid close attention to the relational dimensions of their interactions with hospice patients and their families, and we tended to do so intuitively. During their interviews with me, the volunteers often had to account for these intersubjective processes, articulating how they interpreted their patients' behavior, or what they understood certain behaviors to mean. For example, Emilia's patient with dementia never remembered Emilia's name, but she showed signs that she enjoyed Emilia's company. When Emilia was later confronted with this same patient's family when she was dying, she again had to interpret the nonverbal signals she was receiving from them, which she did by interpreting what she thought they thought she was saying. We judged the quality and success of our communication with our patients and family members almost exclusively through inferences based on our intersubjective experiences. We also recognized that our hospice patients used their interpretation of implicit messages to judge our intentions. For example, I *knew* when I was starting to feel closer to Dorothy, and I have *no doubt* that she felt a closer connection with me at around the same time. However, it would be impossible for me to account for that belief in a way that is any more concrete than the stories I have already told. The patterns that governed the interactions in all the volunteers' stories were co-constructed between the volunteers and their patients and evolved through communication. Every volunteer–patient relationship was a unique creation of the individuals involved.

My observations about the role of intersubjectivity apply generally to close relationships. However, context-specific constraints also influenced intersubjective processes within the volunteer–patient relationship in ways that do not translate to relationships outside hospice. So far, my discussion of intersubjectivity has addressed hospice-as-experienced, but the volunteers also performed their role within the context of hospice-as-organization. Thus, as volunteers, we had to respect our patients' privacy and autonomy to an extent that a friend or family member would not. Sarah illustrated the difference very well when she said, "my Mom jokes about the fact that somehow I can keep my opinions completely shut off with my patient, but with nobody else." Moreover, hospice volunteers cannot always ask questions directly when they want to check their perception of a situation. For example, when Dorothy experienced her first spell, I turned to the hospice nurse for answers, rather than questioning Dorothy or her daughter Terry. When Tom's patient complained that the nursing home had not provided him with a toothbrush, Tom discovered that he had been provided with many, only to lose them. Tom did not confront his patient with this information, because he felt it would violate their relationship.

Additional challenges to open communication arise when the patient's illness involves physical or mental problems related to communication—as with Chris's and Emilia's patients—or when the patient is introverted. In these instances, the volunteers may feel that they should not talk explicitly about their relationship with the patient. It may not be useful to directly ask a patient, "How do you feel about me?" or worse, "What are you thinking?" Rather, as volunteers, we are likely to improvise based on our sense of what's going on at the present moment. Referring to jazz improvisation, Hatch (1999) states, "the best listening and responding involves noticing how others are listening and responding to you" (p. 80). Hatch's observation about how improvisation is contingent upon effective listening efficiently encapsulates the multiple levels of perception expressed in the volunteers' stories of communicating with our patients. Not only do we listen to them listening to us; we also listen to ourselves listening to them listening to us.

To review my discussion of volunteer–patient communication so far, I have described our conversation in terms of the relative absence of talk about death, and focused on intersubjectivity as central to the development and maintenance of volunteer–patient relationships. In both discussions, I present a case for characterizing the communication between volunteers and patients as relational and social, rather than individualistic and psychological. As Lawton (2000) suggests, hospice recognizes "a mutually affecting blend of physical, emotional, social, and spiritual concerns; a conception which both reflects and reinforces a relational, intersubjective notion of the person/self" (p. 159).

As a final comment on the supposed over-reliance on discourse in hospice (Seale, 1998), I suggest that one of the enduring habits of our language is mistakenly to equate communication with talking. A research question such as "How do volunteers communicate with people who are dying?" might appear to require an answer that discusses talking or conversation. However, the stories in this book demonstrate that as we learned how to *be with* our patients, our communication traveled along unexpected and in many ways unremarkable paths, via the shared performance of mundane activities. Doing things with each other became an important means of connecting and building a relationship, an idea with which I conclude this chapter.

FINDING MAGIC IN THE MUNDANE

Throughout the stories in this book, numerous moments are illuminated in which the volunteer and patient connect with each other and take on the feeling of an "us." Many of these magical moments seem to involve what most people would consider highly ordinary or mundane activities. The volunteers' stories revealed how each of them discovered characteristics that made a patient unique, and how they valued the activities, places, or objects that the patient valued. For Dorothy and me, that meant weekly trips to the Crossroads Diner. Emilia would wheel her first patient around the nursing home in search of the family. For Tom, who grew up as a "city kid" in New York and Los Angeles, it involved doing something that meant the world to his patient but was totally foreign to him. Tom was inspired to seek out the prettiest photographs of flowers that he could find and bring them to fill his patient's empty notice board. It is impossible to translate what that gesture meant to his patient, but the story speaks volumes for the magical connection that Tom established with her that night.

Though Shyanne was endowed with many of the trappings of status and privilege—a wealthy family, advanced education, a professional career—she became a student to her patient and found a connection by learning from her patient how to cook squash. Shyanne's story about making squash with Clarice is one of my favorite moments from the research; it stays in my mind as an emblem of the entire volunteer–patient project. Shyanne was willing to adopt the role of student and accept Clarice's pearls of wisdom. Cooking squash together was obviously a meaningful ritual in the emerging relationship between them. When I met Shyanne for our second interview, I recalled this story, and it enriched Shyanne's account of why she elected to become Clarice's health care surrogate, fighting hard to make sure Clarice's pain was addressed. The narrative detail of smuggling apple pies into the ALF dynamically illustrates the connection that Clarice and Shyanne shared. One might have expected Shyanne and Clarice to have difficulty bonding, considering their differences, yet Shyanne, ever self-reflexive about the impact of differences on her relationship with her patient, told me "We instantly connected because we left out all the bullshit and just connected on a human level."

By inviting our patients to share their lives, histories, wisdom, and ideas with us—often putting aside our own preferences in favor of theirs—we did more than send a message that they were valued as human beings; we recognized and embraced the value of being with them and sharing time with them. The content of the activities we shared was less important than the mutuality of giving and receiving, which occurred without fanfare, in all kinds of activities and nonactivities. The "magic" that happens in these moments speaks to the essence of dialogue in the Buberian sense:

> When two men converse together, the psychological is certainly an important part of the situation, as each listens and each prepares to speak. Yet this is only the hidden accompaniment to the conversation itself, the phonetic event fraught with meaning, whose meaning is to be found neither in one of the two partners nor in both together, but only in their dialogue itself, in this "between" which they live together. (Buber, 1988, p. 65)

For the volunteers, the meaningful "between" emerged through interaction in its broadest sense, and in the recognition that our very presence in our patients' lives was inherently significant. Hospice volunteering taught us about what it means to be human and allowed our patients to remain as fully human as possible to the end of life.

The stories in this book provide insight into the experience of communicating with and *being with* hospice patients at the end of their lives. Through their experiences, the volunteers transitioned from a perspective of idealism, through criticism of themselves and hospice-as-organization, to a more realistic and balanced understanding of hospice volunteer work. Despite the primary reason for the volunteers' presence in their patients' lives—that their patients were determined by hospice to be dying—open discussions about death and dying were rare between volunteers and patients. Instead, rather than simply giving back something of themselves in a one-way transaction, their experiences often involved reciprocity and mutuality to an unexpected degree. The relationships between volunteers and patients emerged over time as they participated in mundane activities and allowed magical moments of connection to appear spontaneously in the in between.

In conclusion, having experienced the relational and dialogic quality of the volunteer–patient relationship, I resist the characterization of hospice as inherently individualistic and psychological. I also believe that those who criticize the philosophy of "living until death" (Byock, 1997; Kübler-Ross, 1986) are not sufficiently taking into account hospice-as-experienced by the volunteers and patients. Although hos-pice-as-philosophy may appear individualistic because it is patient–centered, and psychological because it advocates a *meaningful* death, hospice-as-experienced is clearly relational. The volunteers' sto-ries are a testament to the power of *being with* someone who is dying. They illustrate what it was like to appreciate the present moment, to ac-cept the gifts that our patients gave to us, and to allow ourselves to be changed by the experience. In the final section, I offer a personal account of what this change has meant to me.

A PERSONAL STATEMENT

Because the meanings and insights of this book rely so much on stories, and particularly on my own story, I conclude with a personal statement about what this research meant to me. I undertook both hospice volun-teering and this study of hospice because I recognized within my own experience a wider cultural pattern of fearing thoughts of death, and consequently, avoiding people who are dying. As I look back on the liv-ing and the writing of these stories, I see the changes that have been wrought within my way of being through the hospice experience. Through my relationship with Dorothy, and talking with the other vol-unteers, I learned that hospice patients and volunteers establish inti-mate connections, despite obvious constraints on their relationship. The volunteers and patients often shared limited information with each other; they generally did not integrate their lives beyond hospice visits; in some cases, they shared no *meaningful* interaction because the pa-tients could not speak. Nevertheless, intimacy and connection grew through the commitment to *be there* for each other, and through ordinary moments of sharing activities such as eating together, watching televi-sion, or sitting in silence.

I have often overlooked and undervalued mundane activities in inti-mate relationships. I have tended, instead, to look for indications that a relationship is meaningful by seeking more overt evidence such as self-disclosure, expressions of affection, and profound or emotional conversations. My relationship with Dorothy taught me that I could connect with someone whom I hardly know, simply by being there and being willing to let it happen. Rather than sharing deep conversations or emotional revelations, I realized that the intimacy between Dorothy and me was based in relatively ordinary activities and interactions. What made our communication extraordinary was that we were to-gether while Dorothy was nearing the end of her life; we created a new relationship at a time when Dorothy's life consisted mostly of loss. In the past, my fear of dying and its associated losses presented an intrac-table obstacle to my communication with my grandmother and aunt.

When I began volunteering, I feared that I would be similarly challenged in my relationship with a hospice patient. However, because Dorothy's terminal prognosis was a prerequisite for our relationship, the fact that she was dying seemed to fade into the background as I concentrated on trying to get to know her. Later, once we became more comfortable with each other, Dorothy's illness and approaching death generated a feeling of intimacy and *immediacy*. Death and dying were not the focus of the relationship; nor were they an impediment to connection and intimacy. Rather, the simple activities that Dorothy and I enjoyed together were made more significant because I recognized that I was sharing the last weeks and days of her life. I was only able to appreciate my visits with Dorothy once I overcame my preconceived ideas about what I could do to support Dorothy at the end of her life.

The lessons I learned through hospice volunteering required a stripping away of my customary habits of being with other people, rather than learning a series of concepts or acquiring a set of skills. Dorothy did not care about my level of education, what I did for a living, or where I came from. What ultimately mattered in my relationship with her was the kind of person I was, the interest I showed in her, and my commitment to *being there* to share her life. At first, this was difficult for me, partly because it was unfamiliar, and partly because I wasn't sure who I was without the traits that I valued most in myself. Being with Dorothy taught me to release my compulsion to anticipate and control interactions in which I feel unsure of myself. The key to *being with* Dorothy lay in allowing the relationship to reveal itself, learning to improvise and respond spontaneously to each other in the moment. Eventually, I enjoyed simply being with Dorothy in whatever context or condition eventuated. In the end, this meant that I was able to sit with her in silence the day before she died—something I found hard to imagine only a year earlier. In presenting these lessons, I do not presume that they will apply in the same way to all end-of-life situations or relationships. However, I do recognize them as a kind of antidote to the particular fears that I experienced when I faced becoming a volunteer.

I have also learned valuable lessons about how hospice as an organization is perceived by the volunteers. The volunteer training program did not encompass information about the history of the hospice movement, its relationship to Medicare and Medicaid, or the professional organizations that are responsible for hospice accreditation and oversight. Although these aspects of hospice may appear to have little to do with the work of the volunteers, in the volunteers' stories, there were several moments and events that indicated confusion about the rules and philosophy of the organization.

The volunteers in my study often wondered about their "place" in the organization, and questioned what they were contributing to the care of the patient. Part of Hannah's concern with her second patient stemmed from her uncertainty about what she was supposed to feel regarding her patient's death, and she looked to the organization for guidelines about what was right. Emilia's and Chris's patients did not interact with them in the ways that they anticipated when they first went through the training. Although she enjoyed her visits, Emilia struggled to understand what her volunteer activities had provided to her first patient who had dementia. In contrast, Chris relied on his own belief in human contact to give meaning to his relationships with uncommunicative patients, but did not realize that his approach bore a close resemblance to hospice philosophies. The confusion that the volunteers experienced and the sense making that they undertook individually regarding their role in the organization could be addressed with more explicit conversations initiated by the hospice trainers and volunteer coordinators.

The concept of social death helped me to understand the role of the volunteer in the broader context of end-of-life care, and it could provide a valuable addition to the conversations that take place within the hospice organization. I believe hospice should encourage further exploration and development of a relational understanding of hospice volunteering, including more emphasis on the concept of social death. Because current Western thinking is saturated with an individualistic understanding of the self, it is difficult to break from the paradigm of autonomy and control in order to re-language what is occurring *between* hospice volunteers and patients. However, I believe it is precisely the *relational practices* of hospice, rather than its *philosophy* of focusing on the patient as an individual, that distinguishes hospice as a humane alternative to medically based conceptions of dying

In addition to questions about hospice goals and philosophy, the volunteers were affected by rules and regulations about which they were not fully informed. In particular, hospice as an organization could examine the impact of patient graduation on the volunteers. The lack of information given to the volunteers about hospice's procedures of reassessment contributed undue stress to some volunteers, and possibly to their patients. In some cases, volunteers would not ask hospice personnel about their patients' appropriateness. Tom was particularly concerned about "blowing the whistle" inadvertently, and facilitating a review that would result in the loss of his patient. Also related to hospice rules and structures, despite my formal reading about hospice, I was caught off guard by the role of the primary care physician in hospice. When Dorothy could not get her medicine promptly the day before she died, I was dismayed that her physician's office held such a key position in the system, and that hospice could do relatively little to address the lack of response. Removing the primary care physician from this central role would require a radical change in the structure of hospice as it currently exists. However, hospice could alleviate some of the stress from physician-related problems by being more forthcoming about the power that physicians hold in the system, and developing options for when a patient is faced with an unsupportive or unresponsive primary care physician.

I started this project feeling deep regrets about the deaths of my great aunt and grandmother, the only elders who were ever a part of my life, and I have struggled to understand the nature of that regret. At first, I thought that I regretted not talking with them about death, particularly in the case of my grandmother, because I believed that I was the person to whom she was most likely to turn. I also longed for more overt expressions of our feelings and the kinds of deathbed revelations that I have witnessed in films and on television. I now understand, however, that I cannot look back and determine what my interactions with my grandmother and great aunt should have been like, any more than I could have controlled those interactions when they occurred. When I applied the lessons of hospice volunteering to my past experiences, I realized that there is only one thing that I regret—not being with them, not giving them my time, not allowing myself to be in the moment when I was there. I cannot say that my relatives and I would have shared any deep insights about life, or even that I would have affected their deaths in any profound way. What I do know is that I could have been present to share those magical moments of connecting in the silence or the simple activities of life, to witness their being and their dying. Had I allowed myself to do that, I would have those moments forever to cherish in my heart and to remember what it was like to share their last days. The gift that hospice and the writing of this book have given me is the confidence that I will approach other losses in my life, the deaths of those I love, and possibly my own death, with greater composure and capacity to surrender—composure to live and act in the present moment, while surrendering to the uncertainties that accompany the end of life.

Appendix

I have published elsewhere what Van Maanen (1988) would a "confessional tale," which provides a behind-the-scenes account of this study (Foster, 2005a). However, because the method and final form of the research may be unfamiliar to many readers, I include some background information in this Appendix and explain what I did and the theoretical assumptions behind it. The two types of stories in the book—the story of my relationship with Dorothy and the stories provided by the other volunteers—were generated from two types of data: ethnographic field notes and in-depth, qualitative interviewing. In the following sections, I frame the study within the practices of narrative ethnography, and then describe specifics of the interviews, analysis, and process of writing the final manuscript.

NARRATIVE ETHNOGRAPHY

In chapter 1, I described the historical emergence of hospice as an attractive alternative (McGrath, 1998) to the traditional biomedical approach to dying because it is individualized, patient and family directed, and it takes into account the patient's physical, emotional, and spiritual well-being. Similar to the philosophy of hospice care, ethnography also encompasses a researcher perspective and a set of goals that are holistic and multidimensional (Lindlof, 1995), with an emphasis on understanding the observed interactions from the perspective of the participants (Denzin, 1997). Ethnographic studies have an established tradition in aging and end of life research (Adelman & Frey, 1997; Diamond, 1992; Lawton, 2000; Myerhoff, 1979; Rubenstein, 2000). Arguing a relationship between ethnographic research and the process of dying, Rubenstein (2000) proposes the concept of embeddedness as "the quality of dying that sees its meaning in the complex panoply of person, condition, setting, culture, social structure, and other life circumstances that influence the end of life" (p. 259). Ethnographic research is also concerned with meaning as embedded in the practices, language, and events of a culture. The term *ethnography* is derived from the Greek words for tribe or race—*ethnos*—and for writing—*graphos*, or *graphein* (Frey, Botan, & Kreps, 2000; Miller-Day, 2004), and thus ethnography implies two integrally related processes. First, it implies detailed observation of a culture or group through field research and formal or informal interviews. Second, it implies meticulous representation of that culture through a written account (Goodall, 2000). The ethnographic writing process is meticulous not so much in the interest of accurately representing an empirical and monolithic reality, but in order to establish ethical and trustworthy relationships among the researcher, those who are the focus of the research, and those who will become the readers of the research (Gergen & Gergen, 2002). Specifically, the ethnographer articulates a research account that preserves relevant details of the study, including the voices of others, while also allowing readers to make their own discoveries and determinations about what is represented.

Although I had spent many months reading about hospice philosophy and practices, in this study the field research began when I first contacted LifePath Hospice in December 2000 and elected to become a volunteer. The training took place at the beginning of 2001, and I continued to volunteer for LifePath Hospice through June 2002. Although it is considerably larger than most other hospice organizations in the United States—according to its fact sheet (LifePath Hospice and Palliative Care, n.d.), in 2003, LifePath programs provided care to 6,274 individuals and their families—LifePath Hospice and Palliative Care was representative of most hospices in the United States both in its structure and the types of patients that it served. This fact may reassure some readers that there is a basis for generalizing the observations that emerged from this study. My purpose as an ethnographic researcher, however, is not to represent all (or even most) experiences of hospice volunteers and patients everywhere. Rather, my purpose is to represent the events, words, and ideas of this place and these people, and to identify and articulate patterns of meaning that would resonate through other contexts and relationships. My extended period of involvement with hospice combined with the interviews provided me with rich data and a meaningful connection to the activities of volunteering. Both the data and this connection allowed me to draw conclusions about what I learned and how this knowledge might assist others to approach communication at the end of life.

Recognizing that stories and storytelling are central to human reasoning (Fisher, 1984, 1985) and to human relationships (Bochner, Ellis,

& Tillmann-Healy, 1997), this study incorporated an emphasis on narrative. Freeman (1997) suggests that experience, language, and narrative are inextricably linked; that is, to understand an event or relationship is to have a story about it. Just as one goal of hospice care is to find meaning at the end of life (Bradshaw, 1996), narrative integrity depends on our ability to make sense of life by recognizing how each aspect of our experience fits into the whole. Because of its unique ability to embrace both specific details of individual life stories and the wider cultural meanings that those stories reveal, the narrative perspective has been widely adopted by health researchers and theorists (Brody, 1987; Frank, 1991, 1995; Harter, Japp, & Beck, 2005; Kleinmann, 1988; Morris, 1998). In hospice, the link between narrative and practices of sense making may be most obvious in the patient's life review or life history (Dunaway, 1996; Ray, 1998; Sellars & Haag, 1998; Usita, Hyman Jr., & Harman, 1998), in which patients recount stories of their past. Many other communicative activities contribute to hospice care by linking a patient's experiences to a larger system of meaning (Sellars & Haag, 1998). As illustrated by the stories in this book, through listening, exchanging looks, holding hands, and being there with patients, hospice volunteers were given opportunities to witness the unfolding of a life story and register its meaning at a most significant time—its end. In this way, the relationships between volunteers and patients themselves constitute meaningful stories (Bochner, et al., 1997). Thus, narrative ethnography is particularly appropriate as a method to interpret and understand interpersonal communication, because the researcher strives to show meaningful interaction, inviting readers to think *with* the narrative and not merely *about* it (Frank, 1995).

Also in the context of end of life research, autobiographical narratives of illness and dying (e.g. Butler & Rosenblum, 1991; Ellis, 1995a; Frank, 1991; Lorde, 1980) provide insights that encompass practical, ethical, and moral concerns (Bochner, 2001). As Coles (1989) suggests, powerful stories tend to work their way into our "idle thoughts" (p. 204), and so affect our way of thinking as well as our way of being in the world. Some clinicians have adopted autobiographical and narrative approaches when writing about end-of-life care, as evidenced by the nursing journals that regularly feature personal stories of nurse–patient interactions in hospice (Ellner, 1997; Faulkner, 1997; Lafferty, 1997; Pattinson, 1998; Ufema, 1998). From the physician's point of view, Byock's (1997) *Dying Well*, and Barnard, Towers, Boston, and Lambrinidou's (2000) *Crossing Over* present evocative, narrative case studies that have been influential in promoting the "good death" as advocated by hospice. In her book *Soon: Tales from Hospice*, novelist and hospice volunteer Mojtabai (1998) presents fictional stories from the patients' points of view based on her experiences on a hospice ward. In *The*

Measure of Our Days, Groopman (1997) presents a series of case studies that illustrate existential insights he gained while caring for patients who face a variety of life-threatening illnesses. These texts are not concerned with representing dying as it is *for everybody,* but rather as it *could be* for many people. Narrative forms "embrace the power of language to create and change the world, to make new and different things possible" (Bochner, 1994, p. 29), and have been instrumental in changing how we are able to die in this culture.

In terms of method, autoethnography (Reed-Danahay, 1997) implies a process of evocative narrative writing, systematic introspection, and theoretical reflection that is grounded in the lived experience of the fieldworker. Thus, a central feature of this book is the subjective account of my journey as a hospice volunteer. As autoethnography, this narrative was generated through a combination of traditional field notes and via a process of what Ellis (1991) has called "systematic sociological introspection." Specifically, as an autoethnographic researcher, my emotions, thoughts, questions, and perceptions about hospice care became a focus of research in and of themselves. As a "vulnerable observer" (Behar, 1996) of hospice work, my subjectivity, empathy, and identification with others were central to the research process, and in the final text of the book. Particularly because I was writing about an emotionally and morally complex subject (Ellis, 1996), an essential part of my process was to identify and reveal my own responses to the story that I was telling. This reflexivity is present throughout the text in both the personal narrative and the interviews with the other volunteers.

My decision to employ an autoethnographic method was also prompted by ethical considerations associated with the hospice context, in which patient and family privacy and autonomy are paramount. Although the research project was reviewed and approved by the Institutional Review Boards of both the University of South Florida and LifePath Hospice and Palliative Care, such approval is merely the formalization of my ongoing efforts to ensure an ethical relationship between me and others who were within the sphere of the study. Some researchers question whether hospice patients should ever be asked to participate in research (Casarett et al., 2001, p. 442) because of the burden it places on the patient to articulate his or her experience. This perspective echoes the criticism that hospice privileges talk as *the* way to create meaning at the end of life (Lawton, 2000; Seale, 1998; Walter, 1994). As an extension of this critique, Seale (1998) specifically targeted research practices of surveying and interviewing hospice patients, because in addition to burdening the patient, these methods perpetuate a paradigm that values rational thought over bodily emotion. Methodologically, autoethnography shifts the focus of inquiry to the researcher and away from those who might traditionally be considered the subjects of research. Therefore, my adoption of narrative autoethnography as a research and writing strategy addresses these concerns in two ways. First, it does not presume the preeminence of psychology, discourse, or even of rational thought. Rather, autoethnography emphasizes the evocation of the physical and emotional experience, and the communication of meaning through unfolding dramatic action rather than isolated examples framed by explanatory concepts (Ellis, 1996). Second, autoethnography presumes that the burden of expression and sense making is on the researcher rather than on the subjects of the research.

Part of the power of narrative ethnography, and autoethnography in particular, lies in its ability to take the reader into a specific scene, to share dialogue, and to reveal the emotions associated with the experience. But my story is also someone else's story (Behar, 1996), and the question of how to respond to the sharedness of stories presents a very real dilemma for me as a writer of autoethnographic research accounts. When I have conducted personal narrative projects in the past, I have addressed the ethical issues associated with writing about others by sharing my stories with them (Foster, 2001, 2002), or including their writing and responses in the final manuscript (Foster, 2000, 2005b). I could not employ the same strategies as I had in the past because that would mean doing exactly what Seale (1998) claimed—namely, I would be placing a burden on Dorothy, my hospice patient, to reflect upon and articulate the meaning of her own dying.

When it came time to write the account of my relationship with Dorothy, I took seriously the responsibility of writing in a way that focused on our interactions and details of her life that were relevant to the story while changing others to protect her privacy and that of her family. My responsibilities in this regard were different from those of the volunteers I interviewed, because the demands of writing an autoethnographic narrative mean that I offer details of the people in the story, I give them voice and characterize them in a way that invites greater scrutiny than in the volunteers' interviews. Because I valued the times I spent with Dorothy, I experienced conflicting desires to protect these moments by keeping them private and to honor them by sharing them with others. Thankfully, narrative theorists have turned our attention away from facts and toward meanings (Bochner, 2001). This means that the objective for the narrative researcher is to create "narratives that simulate reality, applying the imaginative power of literary, dramatic, and poetic forms to create the effect of reality, a convincing likeness to life as it is sensed, felt, and lived" (Bochner, Ellis, & Tillmann-Healy, 1998, p. 42). My goal in writing this personal narrative was similarly aimed at turning away from the facts of Dorothy's life and toward the meaningful events that stuck with me as I reflected on the months that I spent with her. Ellis (1996) describes going through a similar process when writing certain parts of her book *Final Negotiations*. She writes, "I worked constantly to find a balance between honest writing and good sense, between portraying life as intimately as I could and protecting my relationships with characters in the story and with my readers" (Ellis, 1996, p. 162). With these goals in mind, I wrote a story that reveals an emerging relationship with Dorothy, the everyday details of our weekly visits, and the role that the many facets of communication played in our evolving relationship.

ETHNOGRAPHIC INTERVIEWING

I conducted interviews in order to record other volunteers' stories and also to engage them in the process of reflecting on the meaning of communication and relationships at the end of life. By listening to the stories of other volunteers, I was able to capture and present a wider variety of experiences and insights into the volunteer–patient relationship. I conducted three rounds of interviews—the first was 1 month after graduation in March 2001, the second 6 months later in July and August of 2001, and the third 6 months after that in January and February 2002.

On the night of our graduation, 12 volunteers from the training group expressed an interest in the study. When I called to invite them to complete the first interview, of those 12, 1 expressed an interest in being interviewed later and 2 did not respond to my calls. In the first round, I conducted face-to-face interviews with 9 volunteers. For the second round of interviews, I followed up with the 9 volunteers who had been interviewed during the first round, as well as the volunteer who had been interested but unable to participate in the first round. Of the 10 I contacted, 1 had moved to a different state and the 2 others did not return my calls. At the end of this second round, 6 of the participants had taken part in two interviews, and these 6 became the focus of the volunteer stories presented in this book. Although I tried initially to incorporate the interviews of all participants, the amount of material and the number of different "characters" threatened the coherence of the narrative; thus, it was necessary to be more selective than I originally intended.

For the third round of interviews, I had planned to conduct one or, at most, two group discussions, bringing the participants together to reflect upon the first year of volunteering. I wanted to do this in part because most of the participants had expressed an interest in finding out about the other volunteers, and I also felt it would help me to synthesize the range of experiences and stories into a jointly constructed review of the year. However, the logistics of bringing about such a meeting became extremely complicated and, in the end, the third round of interviews included five meetings involving two group and three individual interviews. Having a range of interview contexts made it difficult to compose a coherent narrative for Part III of the book. However, I decided to persist and for chapter 10 included statements derived from the interview material from the third round. These stories provide a sense of how we looked back over the year, perceived our experiences, and retrospectively connected our experiences to thoughts about the future.

Throughout the study, the style of the interviews was interactive (Ellis & Berger, 2002; Ellis, Kiesinger, & Tillmann-Healy, 1997), because we collaboratively made sense of our hospice experiences, what they meant to us, and what we understood to be our role as volunteers. As demonstrated by the dialogues in the book, in many cases the other volunteers shared stories and asked questions that helped me to frame or reframe my experiences with Dorothy. In accordance with standards for this type of interview, I kept the length and progress of the interviews open-ended. With the exception of the two group discussions in the third round of interviews, which ran for more than 2 hours, each interview lasted between 60 and 90 minutes. During the interviews I concentrated on asking open-ended questions to elicit storytelling (Holloway & Jefferson, 2000), probing the volunteers' interpretations of their experience, as well as disclosing my own experiences. I often employed a two-part question format, which was intended to invite the respondent into my thinking process, and elicit more emotional and narratively-framed responses.

Before the first round of interviews, I informed the participants that the interviews would be tape-recorded and transcribed, and the participants provided consent both verbally and by signing a standard Adult Informed Consent form. In addition to the consent forms, each participant also completed a form in which they provided a pseudonym. Before each interview, I verbally assured the volunteers that I would change the real names of patients they mentioned, and this was also one of the conditions of confidentiality outlined on the consent form. The use of pseudonyms for the participants was offered for their anonymity in the publication as well as to provide an additional level of confidentiality for the patients who were characterized in their stories. At their own request, 2 participants are referred to by their real names, and the name LifePath Hospice and Palliative Care is used with the consent of the director of education and the director of research at LifePath.

Two goals guided my treatment of the interview material as data. I wanted to (a) sustain close attention to the voices of the participants rather than a transcript, and (b) preserve a sense of the context in which the interviews occurred. Both goals were related to my understanding of the interview as a "dialogic world of unique meaning and experience" that should be treated as a whole (Denzin, 1997, p. 38). I felt comfortable lifting examples, expressions, and stories from their context in the theoretical reflections, but only after presenting the discovery process that occurred in collaboration with the other volunteers. Therefore, I faced the challenge of translating the interviews as experienced into evocative written dialogues.

The first stage of the translation process involved transcribing the interview tapes. In order to both retain the voice recordings as my primary source of data and to begin the process of generating a written dialogue, I combined Yow's (1994) oral history method with a detailed transcription process, generating indexed transcripts that allowed me to access the corresponding portions of the tape recordings. The detailed transcription process made me intimately acquainted with the content of the interviews, and the indexing gave me easy access to the spoken word once I began the second stage of translation. The average length of the transcripts from the first two rounds of interviews was 22 single-spaced pages for each participant; the shortest was 12 pages, and the longest was 27 pages. The second stage of translation involved distilling the content of the interviews into relatively brief, coherent, and memorable narratives. I accomplished this through multiple passes through the interviews, first by generally cleaning up the dialogue (retaining only significant hesitations and repetitions), and then by searching for the clearest expression of an idea or story. I accepted the responsibility of interpreting what the volunteers intended to say, and the degree of intervention or editing varied greatly among the volunteers. I continually listened to the tapes throughout this process in order to get a sense of the volunteers' meanings, which were not always evident in the words as they appeared on the raw transcripts. By comparing the word counts of the transcripts and their corresponding stories in the book manuscript, I later found that I selected an average of less than 20% of each interview.

My translation of the transcribed interviews was also guided by a desire to achieve thematic focus across the interviews. Kleinman, Copp, and Henderson (1997) point out that fieldwork and analysis are not separate processes despite the way they are traditionally presented in social scientific research accounts. As I translated the interview data, I was also initiating a process of analysis whereby I identified themes that recurred across and within the various interviews as well as within my own experience. Throughout the translation process, I returned to my primary interest in communication and the volunteer–patient relationship. If I were to operationalize this as a criterion by which I selected portions of the interviews, I would say that I looked for specific descriptions of what the volunteers did, what they said, and what they felt when visiting and communicating with their patients. These themes became the foundation of the theoretical reflections throughout the book.

The third round of interviews presented a difficult narrative challenge. Not only were some of these interviews conducted through group discussion, which meant that the conversation differed in rhythm and tone from the earlier interviews, but they also varied greatly in length, with the shortest individual interview lasting for 45 minutes and the group discussions over 2 hours. At this point, given the development of dialogues from the interviews and my own story, my attention was drawn to the needs of the reader and the story that had been unfolding. In chapter 10, where the third round of interviews is presented, my goals were to show the reader where each volunteer's story had gone, to present their reflections on the meaning of their experiences, and to foreshadow the analysis in chapter 11. This was the most difficult of all the translations, because I wanted to demonstrate the resonance across the interviews but did not have a true focus group dialogue to work from. The compromise I made was to select lengthy quotes from the transcripts and weave them together thematically, with interjections and explanations to guide the reader. Although this form does not reach the fluidity of a true dialogue, I believe that the stories presented in Parts II and III were better served by presenting the voices in parallel reflections rather than in a series of monologues or the lengthier form of the interviews that preceded them. The multiple voices also allowed certain themes to emerge more sharply into focus without necessarily tying off and smoothing over every thread, or answering every question raised by the study.

I would like to make one final statement in relation to the methods used in this study. Although many researchers, particularly in the social sciences, are familiar with equating rigor with experimental control, empirical measurement, and the distanced stance of observation, ethnography demands a rigor that bears much in common with the rigor of volunteering. Specifically, ethnography demands commitment not just to the pursuit of answering a research question, but to the people and contexts that may be affected by one's pursuit of answers. Furthermore, the practice of narrative ethnography, like hospice volunteering, demands that researchers be willing to bring all necessary resources to the task at hand including their creativity, emotions, empathy, critical insight, and sometimes a willingness to follow their own hearts in defiance of others' expectations. The researcher becomes the instrument through which others may come to know an unfamiliar world or to see a familiar world through new eyes. By electing to study communication at the end of life in this way, I invite others to view the process of understanding as *caring* and not just reading, as *being* and not just thinking, and as an act of engaging with the world and endeavoring to make a difference.

References

Adelman, M. B., & Frey, L. R. (1997). *The fragile community: Living together with AIDS*. Mahwah, NJ: Lawrence Erlbaum Associates.

Albom, M. (1997). *Tuesdays with Morrie: An old man, a young man, and life's greatest lesson*. New York: Doubleday.

Anderson, R., & Cissna, K. N. (1997). *The Martin Buber–Carl Rogers dialogue: A new transcript with commentary*. Albany: State University of New York.

Archer, M. S. (1995). *Realist social theory: A morphogenetic approach*. Cambridge, UK: Cambridge University.

Baglia, J. (2005). *The Viagra ad venture: Masculinity, media, and the performance of sexual health*. New York: Lang.

Barbalet, J. M. (1998). *Emotion, social theory, and social structure*. Cambridge, UK: Cambridge University.

Barnard, D., Towers, A., Boston, P., & Lambrinidou, Y. (2000). *Crossing over: Narratives of palliative care*. New York: Oxford University Press.

Barnes, M. K., & Duck, S. (1994). Everyday communicative contexts for social support. In B. R. Burleson, T. L. Albrecht, & I. G. Sarason (Eds.), *Communication of social support: Messages, interactions, relationships, and community* (pp. 175–194). Thousand Oaks, CA: Sage.

Bateson, G. (1951). Information and codification: A philosophical approach. In J. Reusch & G. Bateson (Eds.), *Communication: The social matrix of psychiatry* (pp. 168–211). New York: Norton.

Baxter, L. A., & Montgomery, B. M. (1996). *Relating: Dialogues and dialectics*. New York: Guilford.

Becker, E. (1997). *The denial of death*. New York: Free Press.

Behar, R. (1996). *The vulnerable observer*. Boston: Beacon.

Bennahum, D. A. (1996). The historical development of hospice and palliative care. In D. C. Sheehan & W. B. Forman (Eds.), *Hospice and palliative care: Concepts and practice* (pp. 1–10). London: Jones and Bartlett.

Berger, C. R., & Calabrese, R. J. (1975). Some explorations in initial interaction and beyond: Toward a developmental theory of interpersonal communication. *Human Communication Research, 1*, 99–112.

Berger, P. L., & Luckmann, T. (1967). *The social construction of reality: A treatise in the sociology of knowledge*. Garden City, NY: Anchor.

Bochner, A. P. (1994). Perspectives on inquiry II: Theories and stories. In M. Knapp & G. R. Miller (Eds.), *Handbook of interpersonal communication* (2nd ed.) (pp. 21–41). Thousand Oaks, CA: Sage.

Bochner, A. P. (1995). On the efficacy of openness in close relationships. In M. V. Redmond (Ed.), *Interpersonal communication: Readings in theory and research* (pp. 256–268). Fort Worth, TX: Harcourt Brace.

Bochner, A. P. (2001). Narrative's virtues. *Qualitative Inquiry, 7*, 131–157.

Bochner, A. P., Ellis, C., & Tillmann-Healy, L. M. (1997). Relationships as stories. In S. Duck (Ed.), *Handbook of personal relationships* (2nd ed.) (pp. 308 – 324). New York: Wiley.

Bochner, A. P., Ellis, C., & Tillmann-Healy, L. (1998). Mucking around looking for truth. In B. M. Montgomery & L. A. Baxter (Eds.), *Dialectical approaches to studying personal relationships* (pp. 41–62). Mahwah, NJ: Lawrence Erlbaum Associates.

Bradley, E. H., Fried, T. R., Kasl, S. V., & Idler, E. (2000). Quality-of-life trajectories of elders in the end of life. *Annual Review of Gerontology and Geriatrics, 20*, 66–96.

Bradshaw, A. (1996). The spiritual dimension of hospice: The secularization of an ideal. *Social Science and Medicine, 43*, 409–419.

Brand, D. (1988, September 5). Dying with dignity: Cicely Saunders started the modern hospice movement in London 21 years ago. *Time, 132*(10), 56–58.

Brilhart, J. K., & Galanes, G. J. (1995). *Effective group discussion* (8th ed.). Madison, WI: Brown and Benchmark.

Brody, H. (1987). *Stories of sickness.* New Haven, CT: Yale University Press.

Brook, P. (1968). *The empty space.* New York: Atheneum.

Bruner, J. (1986). *Actual minds, possible worlds.* Cambridge, MA: Harvard University.

Buber, M. (1970). *I and Thou* (W. Kaufmann, Trans.). New York: Scribner.

Buber, M. (1988). *The knowledge of man: Selected essays.* M. Friedman (Ed.) (Revised ed.). Atlantic Highlands, NJ: Humanities Press International. (Original work published 1965)

Burleson, B. R., Albrecht, T. L., & Sarason, I. G. (Eds.). (1994). *Communication of social support: Messages, interactions, relationships, and community.* Thousand Oaks, CA: Sage.

Butler, R. N., Burt, R., Foley, K. M., Morris, J., & Morrison, R. S. (1996). A peaceful death: How to manage pain and provide quality care (part 2). *Geriatrics, 51*(6), 32–37.

Butler, S., & Rosenblum, B. (1991). *Cancer in two voices.* Duluth, MN: Spinsters Ink.

Byock, I. (1997). *Dying well: Peace and possibilities at the end of life.* New York: Riverhead.

Callanan, M., & Kelley, P. (1992). *Final gifts: Understanding the special awareness, needs, and communications of the dying.* New York: Simon and Schuster.

Carey, J. (1992). *Communication and culture: Essays on media and society.* New York: Routledge.

Carr, W. F. (1995). Spiritual pain and healing in the hospice. *America, 173*(4), 26–29.

Casarett, D., Ferrell, B., Kirschling, J., Levetown, M., Merriman, M. P., Ramey, M., et al. (2001). NHCPO task force statement on the ethics of hospice participation in research. *Journal of Palliative Medicine, 4*, 441–449.

Coles, R. (1989). *The call of stories: Teaching and the moral imagination.* Boston: Houghton Mifflin.

Conley, V. M. (2000, January). *Eat dessert first.* Paper presented at the annual Couch–Stone Symposium on Ethnography for the 21st Century, St. Petersburg, FL.

Conley, V. M. (2001, November). *The role of values of terminally ill patients' and caregivers' behaviors*. Paper presented at the annual meeting of the National Communication Association, Atlanta, GA.

Connor, S. R. (1998). *Hospice: Practice, pitfalls, and promise*. Washington, DC: Taylor and Francis.

Conville, R. L. (1998). Telling stories: Dialectics of relational transition. In B. M. Montgomery & L. A. Baxter (Eds.), *Dialectical approaches to studying personal relationships* (pp. 17–40). Mahwah, NJ: Lawrence Erlbaum Associates.

Coupland, J., & Gwyn, R. (Eds.) (2003). *Discourse, the body, and identity*. Basingstoke, UK: Palgrave Macmillan.

Denzin, N. K. (1997). *Interpretive ethnography: Ethnographic practices for the 21st century*. Thousand Oaks, CA: Sage.

Diamond, T. (1992). *Making gray gold: Narratives of nursing home care*. Chicago, IL: University of Chicago.

Duck, S. (1990). Relationships as unfinished business: Out of the frying pan and into the 1990s. *Journal of Social and Personal Relationships, 7*, 5–28.

Dunaway, D. K. (1996). Introduction: The interdisciplinarity of oral history. In D. K. Dunaway & W. K. Baum (Eds.), *Oral history: An interdisciplinary anthology* (2nd ed.) (pp. 7–22). Walnut Creek, CA: AltaMira.

Eisenberg, E. M. (1990). Jamming: Transcendence through organizing. *Communication Research, 17*, 139–164.

Ellis, C. (1991). Sociological introspection and emotional experience. *Symbolic Interaction, 14*, 23–50.

Ellis, C. (1995a). *Final negotiations: A story of love, loss, and chronic illness*. Philadelphia: Temple University.

Ellis, C. (1995b). Speaking of dying: An ethnographic short story. *Symbolic Interaction, 18*, 73–81.

Ellis, C. (1996). On the demands of truthfulness in writing personal loss narratives. *Journal of Personal and Interpersonal Loss, 1*, 151–177.

Ellis, C., & Berger, L. (2002). Their story/my story/our story: Including the researcher's experience in interview research. In J. F. Gubrium & J. A. Holstein (Eds.), *Handbook of interview research: Context and method* (pp. 847–876). Thousand Oaks, CA: Sage.

Ellis, C., & Bochner, A. P. (2000). Autoethnography, personal narrative, reflexivity: Researcher as subject. In N. K. Denzin & Y. S. Lincoln (Eds.), *The handbook of qualitative research* (2nd ed.) (pp. 733–768). Thousand Oaks, CA: Sage.

Ellis, C., Kiesinger, C., & Tillmann-Healy, L. (1997). Interactive interviewing: Talking about emotional experience. In R. Hertz (Ed.), *Reflexivity and voice* (pp. 119–149). Thousand Oaks, CA: Sage.

Ellner, L. R. (1997). What Grandma Clara wanted: Death with dignity. *American Journal of Nursing, 97*(8), 51.

Esslin, M. (1987). *The field of drama: How the signs and meanings of drama create meaning on stage and screen*. London: Methuen.

Faulkner, K. W. (1997). Talking about death with a dying child. *American Journal of Nursing, 97*(6), 64–67.

Fisher, W. (1985). The narrative paradigm: An elaboration. *Journal of Communication, 35*, 74–89.

Fisher, W. R. (1984). Narration as human communication paradigm: The case for public moral argument. *Communication Monographs, 51*, 1–22.

Foster, E. (2000). Reaching out, reaching in, and holding on: Friendship, attempted suicide, and recovery. *American Communication Association Journal, 2*(2). Available from http://www.americancomm.org/~aca/acjdata/vol2/Iss1/essays/foster.htm

Foster, E. (2001). Hurricanes: A narrative of conflict cycles in a distressed marriage. *Studies in Symbolic Interaction, 24,* 171–194.

Foster, E. (2002). Storm tracking: Scenes of marital disintegration. *Qualitative Inquiry, 8,* 804–819.

Foster, E. (2005a). Communication at the end of life: Volunteer–patient relationships in hospice. In S. H. Priest (Ed.) *Communication impact: Designing research that matters* (pp. 143–157). Lanham, MD: Rowman and Littlefield.

Foster, E. (2005b). Desiring dialectical discourse: A feminist ponders the transition to motherhood. *Women's Studies in Communication, 28,* 57–83.

Frank, A. W. (1991). *At the will of the body: Reflections on illness.* New York: Houghton Mifflin.

Frank, A. W. (1995). *The wounded storyteller: Body, illness, and ethics.* Chicago: University of Chicago.

Freeman, M. (1997). Death, narrative integrity, and the radical challenge of self-understanding: A reading of Tolstoy's "The Death of Ivan Illich." *Ageing and Society, 17,* 373–397.

Frey, L. R., Botan, C. H., & Kreps, G. L. (2000). *Investigating communication: An introduction to research methods* (2nd ed.). Boston: Allyn & Bacon.

Friedrich, M. J. (1999). Hospice care in the United States: A conversation with Florence Wald. *Journal of the American Medical Association, 281,* 1683–1684.

Geist-Martin, P., Ray, E. B., & Sharf, B. F. (2003). *Communicating health: Personal, cultural, and political complexities.* Belmont, CA: Wadsworth.

Gergen, K. J. (1994). *Realities and relationships: Soundings in social construction.* Cambridge, MA: Harvard University.

Gergen, M. M., & Gergen, K. J. (2002). Ethnographic representation as relationship. In A. P. Bochner & C. Ellis (Eds.), *Ethnographically speaking: Autoethnography, literature, & aesthetics* (pp. 11–33). Walnut Creek, CA: AltaMira.

Giddens, A. (1984). *The constitution of society: Outline of the theory of structuration.* Berkeley: University of California.

Glaser, B. G., & Strauss, A. L. (1965). *Awareness of dying.* Chicago: Aldine.

Glaser, B. G., & Strauss, A. L. (1967). *The discovery of grounded theory: Strategies for qualitative research.* New York: Aldine.

Glaser, B. G., & Strauss, A. L. (1968). *A time for dying.* Chicago: Aldine.

Goffman, E. (1986). *Stigma: Notes on the management of spoiled identity.* New York: Touchstone.

Goodall, H. L., Jr. (2000). *Writing the new ethnography.* Walnut Creek, CA: AltaMira.

Groopman, J. (1997). *The measure of our days: New beginnings at life's end.* New York, NY: Viking.

Gudykunst, W. B., & Kim, Y. Y. (1984). *Communicating with strangers: An approach to intercultural communication.* New York: Random House.

Harter, L. M., Japp, P. M., & Beck, C. S. (Eds.). (2005). *Narratives, health, and healing: Communication theory, research, and practice.* Mahwah, NJ: Lawrence Erlbaum Associates.

Hatch, M. J. (1999). Exploring the empty spaces of organizing: How improvisational jazz helps redescribe organizational structure. *Organization Studies, 20,* 75–100.

Hayslip, B., Jr., & Leon, J. (1992). *Hospice care.* Newbury Park, CA: Sage.

Hickey, J. G. (1999, January 25). A safe haven for the dying?: Reform needed in hospice care. *Insight on the News, 15,* 14.

Holloway, W., & Jefferson, T. (2000). *Doing qualitative research differently: Free association, narrative, and the interview method.* London: Sage.

Hook, C. C., & Mueller, P. S. (2005). The Terry Schiavo saga: The making of a tragedy and lessons learned. *Mayo Clinic Proceedings, 80,* 1449–1460.

Johanson, G. A., & Johanson, I. V. (1996). The core team. In D. C. Sheehan & W. B. Forman (Eds.), *Hospice and palliative care: Concepts and practice* (pp. 31–40). London: Jones and Bartlett.

Jourard, S. (1971). *The transparent self.* New York: Wiley.

Kerby, A. P. (1991). *Narrative and the self.* Bloomington: Indiana University.

Keeley, M. P., & Koenig Kellas, J. (2005). Constructing life and death through final conversation narratives. In L. M. Harter, P. M. Japp, & C. S. Beck (Eds.), *Narratives, health, and healing: Communication theory, research, and practice* (pp. 365–388). Mahwah, NJ: Lawrence Erlbaum Associates.

Kiesinger, C. (1999, August). *The touch, texture, and experience of death: A narrative journey.* Paper presented at the annual meeting of the Society for the Study of Symbolic Interaction, Chicago, IL.

Kiesinger, C. (2001, February). *Portraits of grief.* Paper presented at the annual Couch– Stone Symposium of the Society for the Study of Symbolic Interaction, Miami, FL.

Kleinman, S., Copp, M. A., & Henderson, K. A. (1997). Qualitatively different: Teaching fieldwork to graduate students. *Journal of Contemporary Ethnography, 25,* 469–499.

Kleinmann, A. (1988). *The illness narratives.* New York: Basic Books.

Kübler-Ross, E. (1986). *Death: The final stage of growth.* New York: Simon and Schuster.

Kübler-Ross, E. (1969). *On death and dying.* New York: Macmillan.

Laing, R. D. (1990). *Self and others.* London: Penguin.

Lafferty, C. L. (1997). A parting gift: A simple bed bath would mean so much? *Nursing, 27*(8), 80.

Lawton, J. (2000). *The dying process: Patients' experiences of palliative care.* London: Routledge.

LifePath Hospice and Palliative Care (n.d.). *LifePath Hospice and Palliative Care fact sheet.* Retrieved March 6, 2005 from www.lifepath-hospice.org.

Lindlof, T. R. (1995). *Qualitative communication research methods.* Thousand Oaks, CA: Sage.

Lockhart, C. A., Volk-Craft, B. E., Hamilton, G., Aiken, L. S., & Williams, F. G. (2003). The PhoenixCare Program. *Journal of Palliative Medicine, 6,* 1001–1012.

Lorde, A. (1980). *The cancer journals.* San Francisco: Aunt Lute Books.

McGrath, P. (1998). A spiritual response to the challenge of routinization: A dialogue of discourses in a Buddhist initiated hospice. *Qualitative Health Research, 8,* 801–812.

Martin, S. (2002, June 17 & 24). The death of my father. *The New Yorker, 84,* 86–87.

Miller-Day, M. A. (2004). *Communication among grandmothers, mothers, and daughters: A qualitative study of maternal relationships.* Mahwah, NJ: Lawrence Erlbaum Associates.

Miller, S. C., Mor, V., Gage, M., & Coppola, K. (2000). Hospice and its role in improving end-of-life care. *Annual Review of Gerontology and Geriatrics, 20,* 193–223.

Mojtabai, A. G. (1998). *Soon: Tales from hospice.* Cambridge, MA: Zoland.

Montgomery, B. M., & Baxter, L. A. (Eds.). (1998). *Dialectical approaches to studying personal relationships.* Mahwah, NJ: Lawrence Erlbaum Associates.

Moore, A. (1998, March 2). Hospice care hijacked?: Christian vision versus business considerations. *Christianity Today, 42,* 38–41.

Morris, D. (Producer). (1998). *ABC News Presents: Lessons on living.* [Television broadcast: Interview with Morrie Schwartz by Ted Koppell]. Howell, MI. ABC News.

Morris, D. B. (1998). *Illness and culture in the postmodern age.* Berkeley: University of California.

Myerhoff, B. (1980). *Number our days.* New York: Touchstone.

National Hospice & Palliative Care Organization, (n.d.). *Information Central: Hospice Statistics and Research.* Retrieved March 6, 2005 from www.nhpco.org.

Pattinson, S. (1998). Learning to fly: How a hospice patient and a nurse taught each other about living. *Nursing, 28*(6), 104.

Perry, J. E., Churchill, L. R., & Kirschner, H. S. (2005). The Terry Schiavo case: Legal, ethical, and medical perspectives. *Annals of Internal Medicine, 143,* 744–748.

Public Affairs Television (Producer). (2000). *On Our Own Terms* [Television series]. New York: WNET.

Rawlins, W. K. (1992). *Friendship matters: Communication, dialectics, and the life course.* New York: Aldine de Gruyter.

Ray, R. E. (1998). Introduction: Critical perspectives on the life story. *Journal of Aging Studies, 12,* 101–106.

Reed-Danahay, D. E. (1997). *Auto/ethnography: Rewriting the self and the social.* Oxford, England: Berg.

Richardson, L. (1994). Writing as a method of inquiry. In N. Denzin & Y. Lincoln (Eds.), *Handbook of qualitative inquiry* (pp. 516–529). Thousand Oaks, CA: Sage.

Rogers, E. R., & Escudero, V. (2004). Theoretical foundations. In L. E. Rogers & V. Escudero (Eds.), *Relational communication: An interactional perspective to the study of process and form* (pp. 3–22). Mahwah, NJ: Lawrence Erlbaum Associates.

Rothwell, J. D. (2001). *In mixed company: Small group communication* (4th ed.). Fort Worth, TX: Harcourt.

Rubenstein, R. L. (2000) The ethnography of the end of life: The nursing home and other residential settings. *Annual Review of Gerontology and Geriatrics, 20,* 259–272.

Seale, C. (1998). *Constructing death: The sociology of dying and bereavement.* Cambridge, UK: Cambridge University.

Sellers, C. S., & Haag, B. A. (1998). Spiritual nursing interventions. *Journal of Holistic Nursing, 16,* 338–354.

Shapiro, J. P. (1997, March 24). Death be not swift enough: Fraud fighters begin to probe the expense of hospice care. *U.S. News and World Report, 122*(11), 34–35.

Sontag, S. (1990). *Illness as metaphor; and, AIDS and its metaphors.* New York: Doubleday.

Tedlock, B. (1991). From participant observation to the observation of participation: The emergence of narrative ethnography. *Journal of Anthropological Research, 41,* 69–94.

Tompkins, J. (1996). *A life in school: What the teacher learned.* New York: Addison Wesley Longman.

Turner, V. (1995). *The ritual process: Structure and anti-structure.* Hawthorne, NY: Aldine de Gruyter.

Ufema, J. (1998). Insights on death and dying. *Nursing, 28*(10), 66–67.

Usita, P. M., Hyman, I. E., Jr., & Harman, K. C. (1991). Narrative intentions: Listening to the life stories in Alzheimer's disease. *Journal of Aging Studies, 12,* 185–197.

Van Maanen, J. (1988). *Tales of the field.* Chicago: University of Chicago.

Varela, F. J., Thompson, E., & Rosch, E. (1991). *The embodied mind: Cognitive science and human experience.* Cambridge, MA: MIT.

Walter, T. (1994). *The revival of death.* London: Routledge.

Watzlawick, P., Beavin, J. H., & Jackson, D. D. (1967). *Pragmatics of human communication.* New York: Norton.

Yow, V. (1994). *Recording oral history: A practical guide for social scientists.* Thousand Oaks, CA: Sage.

Author Index

233

Subject Index